Bach Flower Remedies for Dogs

Bach Flower Remedies for Dogs

Martin J. Scott and Gael Mariani

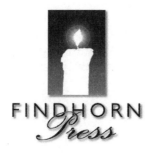

FINDHORN
Press

First published by Findhorn Press 2007

ISBN: 978-1-84409-099-0

British Library Cataloguing-in-Publication Data.
A catalogue record for this book is available from the British Library.

Edited by Jane Engel
Cover design by Damian Keenan
Layout by Pam Bochel
Printed and bound by WS Bookwell, Finland

1 2 3 4 5 6 7 8 9 10 11 12 13 12 11 10 09 08 07

Published by
Findhorn Press
305A The Park,
Findhorn, Forres
Scotland IV36 3TE

Tel 01309 690582
Fax 01309 690036
email: info@findhornpress.com
www.findhornpress.com

Contents

Acknowledgements

The authors wish to express their sincere gratitude to all those who have helped with the long, difficult but always deeply satisfying process of researching the ways that Bach flower remedies and other flower essences can help animals. Special thanks must go to Richard Allport, MRCVS, Patron of the Society for Animal Flower Essence Research; Joanne Vyse-Killa, VN; Carole and Stewart Thornley at the Aricia Dog Training Centre; Julian Barnard; Jonathan Wright, DVM and Melissa Wright; Colin Tennant and Ross McCarthy at the Canine and Feline Behaviour Association; David Cavill, publisher of *Dogs Monthly* magazine; London-based dog trainer Christine Bradley; Erica Bennett at Sheila Harper Canine Education; Sandra Morris, Wales-based canine behaviour consultant; and the many other friends and associates too numerous to list here.

Finally, heartfelt thanks must go to the many dogs and other animals who have proved our wisest and most valuable teachers over the years.

We dedicate this book to the memory of Jessie.

Authors' Preface

The authors have been very involved for several years with Bach flower remedies and their uses in animal care. In 1998 we had the privilege of founding the first organisation in the world to specifically research and explore the ways that flower remedies could benefit animals: the Society for Animal Flower Essence Research (S.A.F.E.R). Operating the Society has been an exciting time and we are very indebted to the many valued associates and helpers who have joined us along the way. S.A.F.E.R has been very fortunate in helping to promote the use of these profoundly effective and safe natural remedies for the benefit of many animals across the world. The tide is turning, and we are now beginning to see more and more use of flower remedies in animal rescue and rehabilitation centres to help the victims of cruelty, neglect and abandonment; in veterinary clinics to aid in the healing process for frightened, stressed or weak animals; in wild animal charity work; compassionate animal training centres; and, last but not least, in the homes of caring and dedicated pet owners everywhere who want to help their animals live a healthier, happier life. Bach flower remedies are truly one of the greatest gifts we have received from nature, and they are one of the greatest gifts we can give to any person we care for – whether that 'person' be a human loved one or a cherished animal friend and companion.

We have written this book for anyone interested in dogs and their welfare, happiness and health. You may know nothing about the Bach remedies, may know a little or may have worked with the remedies for many years. Whatever your involvement with dogs – veterinary science, canine training and behaviour, rescue and rehabilitation, or the dedicated carer wishing to know more about how to improve the life of their canine companion – this book will give you a solid understanding of the many uses of Bach flower remedies in their care.

Foreword

By Julian Barnard

Animals experience a range of emotions in a similar way to human beings. Perhaps that is why we like them as pets. That a dog feels is self evident and those feelings can be intimately bound up with the feelings of their owner. So a skillful practitioner will often see the need to help the person and their pet together. Perhaps, therefore, the title of this book should be *Bach Flower Remedies for Dogs and their People*! For this is a book about much more than prescriptive treatments for canines. In straightforward and practical ways the authors have approached the whole subject of flower therapy. Read it and you will learn about yourself as much as about your dog.

'Dogs should be taught to be emotionally independent...' we are told here and the same thought was in Dr Bach's mind when he spoke out against the way we can interfere with the lives of others. So this subject could be quite a challenge. But it is written about in a caring and approachable way and from the first page elicits the reader's attention and interest. If we can learn how to identify the emotions of our pet then we can learn to identify our own emotions and understand the part they play in our health and wellbeing. It is a book to reread and think about: it is an introduction to many wider issues of science and psychology.

Julian Barnard is widely known as the leading authority on the life and works of Dr Edward Bach. He is the author of many books about the Bach flower remedies, and edited and published the first complete edition of Dr Bach's original writings. He is the Founder and Director of Healing Herbs Ltd, and has lectured on the flower remedies in more than a dozen countries worldwide.

Introduction

Lucky's Story

Lucky, a silver-blue lurcher (a greyhound-type) dog, had lived all his three years in a quiet Welsh village with his carer, Mick. Mick was deeply devoted to his dog and the two would go everywhere together, often seen walking down the street to the butcher where Mick had been collecting his daily meat and bones for his dogs for the past thirty years. Their relationship was one of security, routine and happy companionship.

Until, one day, a spate of dog thefts hit the area. The thieves were targeting greyhound and lurcher-type dogs, intent on re-selling them for illegal hare hunting or 'coursing'. The dog thieves would watch out for such dogs in the street, follow their owners home and wait for an opportunity to strike. Mick was just one of the unlucky people to have their dogs stolen. First thinking that Lucky might have wandered off – though it seemed like strange behaviour from his close companion – he contacted the police, local dog pounds, and a number of animal rescue organisations. But to his growing despair, there was no sign of Lucky anywhere.

Three months later, Lucky was still missing. Mick had all but given up hope of ever finding him, and his heart was broken. Then, one day, a letter appeared in the local newspaper, written by a local farmer. It seemed that a greyhound-type dog was living rough up in the hills, scavenging in the garbage and catching rabbits. The farmer and his family had been leaving food out for the dog, but had been unable to catch him. After reading the letter, Mick contacted the farmer and visited the farm. It wasn't long before the dog showed up. Mick recognised him immediately from his distinguishing marks – it certainly seemed to be Lucky. But was it? The dog didn't show any sign of recognition. It wasn't until, after a whole day of trying to lure the dog into a shed to catch him, that Mick was finally able to confirm that it really was Lucky. He was thinner, filthy and ragged, but he was the same dog right down to the name tag on his collar. How had he ended up on the farm? Had he managed to escape from his captors? It was a mystery, but all Mick cared about was that he'd got his dog back.

That should have been the happy ending to the story, but it was only the start of the real problem. When Mick brought Lucky home to the place where he had spent three happy years, his whole contented life, he screamed, howled, trembled, and wouldn't look at anything or anyone. His whole body and head were pressed against the wall, unable to move and frozen in terror. This was obviously a creature suffering from extreme mental trauma.

Mick was beside himself with distress. Lucky was seen by vets, but although he was emaciated there was nothing physically wrong with him. However, the vets agreed that Lucky was in pain: psychological pain. If the dog didn't improve, Mick faced the prospect of having to have him put to sleep. It seemed cruel to let a dog live in such a state.

This situation went on for a while, until by chance a haggard and careworn Mick mentioned Lucky's state to a local dog groomer, Eryl. Eryl had recently attended a talk given by the directors of S.A.F.E.R, the Society for Animal Flower Essence Research, the authors of this book. The talk had made her interested in using Bach flower remedies for dogs, and she remembered from her notes that there might be something there to help Lucky. She suggested the Bach remedy Star of Bethlehem to Mick. He was sceptical, but he was also desperate. He quickly obtained a small bottle of Star of Bethlehem. Within an hour of giving the first few drops to Lucky, he called Eryl in amazement.

The first reaction to the remedy had come after about twenty minutes, when the expression of terror lifted slightly from Lucky's eyes. He turned away from the wall, and looked at Mick with the beginnings of recognition. After a few more minutes there was a small, but definite, wag of the tail.

Both Eryl and Mick thought it would take many days for Lucky to recover further, but they were happy to be proved wrong. The dog's progress was rapid, and with drops of Star of Bethlehem twice a day it only took a week before he was completely back to his old self. He put the weight back on, his coat regained its former healthy sheen, and they never looked back. Mick never doubted for a second that Dr Bach's Star of Bethlehem was what saved Lucky from chronic trauma and probable euthanasia.

Lucky is just one of thousands of dogs who have benefited, and even had their lives saved, by these simple yet profound remedies.

Chapter One

What are the Bach Flower Remedies?

If you have picked up this book, you may already be familiar with this system of natural therapy pioneered by Dr Edward Bach (1886–1936). For those less familiar, the Bach flower remedies are a range of liquid remedies prepared from wild flowers. Their purpose is mainly in helping to heal negative emotional states: that is to say, states of mind and mood that cause suffering, or which are the result of suffering. These states of mind include emotions like sadness and despair, fear and anxiety, hostility and defensiveness, and the effects of emotional trauma past and present. The remedies come in liquid form, and are generally taken orally – although there are various other ways to use them, which we will be discussing in this book. They are 100% safe, inexpensive and widely available throughout the world. Animals respond to them particularly well, sometimes showing signs of improvement within minutes!

The Bach flower remedies are a strange paradox. They represent a fabulous technology of nature whose workings on living organisms are still something of a mystery to our crude human science. Yet for all its depth this natural healing resource is almost absurdly simple to use – so simple, in fact, that anyone can use the remedies without any previous study or knowledge. The results speak for themselves. For over seventy years now, this unassuming collection of gentle but powerful remedies has been quietly changing the lives of millions of people – and animals – across the world.

Many books have been written about the wide potential of Bach flower remedies to help with the problems we humans are so prone to. In this book we are going to shift the focus a little to look at how they can be used to help a fellow species we have brought into our human world: the dog, in all its many shapes and sizes. We'll examine the many ways that Bach remedies can change the lives of dogs that are suffering from problems of the emotions, such as fear or stress or psychological tension stemming from past maltreatment.

Amongst plant-based natural remedies (herbs, essential oils, homeopathy etc.) Bach flower remedies occupy a special and unique place, not just because they are prepared like no other type of remedy but also because they are so simple to learn and use. It isn't possible to cause any problems with them, and any 'mistakes' you make by choosing an inappropriate remedy can easily and quickly be fixed simply by making a different choice and trying again. Flower remedies are a very forgiving subject to learn for the beginner. What this means is that even if you have never used them before, the information in this book will be more than enough to get you started using Bach flower remedies effectively to help the lives of dogs or any other suffering creature, including humans. In a world where it seems so easy to do the wrong thing even with the best of intentions, Bach remedies seem to offer the impossible: something that can only do good. That's the beautiful reality of this system of therapy.

The life and legacy of Dr Edward Bach

Although it has its origins in history stretching back hundreds and possibly thousands of years, Dr Edward Bach is the person generally credited with the invention of the science of flower remedies. He was an English physician who gradually became increasingly disenchanted with conventional medical practice, and finally broke away, six years before his death, to develop a collection of special liquid-based remedies that were to become famous as the Bach Flower Remedies.

Edward Bach was an extremely caring and kind man who was deeply committed to relieving suffering in whatever way he could. His childhood love of nature, of plants and animals, was to be a guiding force throughout his medical career.

Early medical career

Bach qualified as a doctor in 1912. His health was never strong, and he was turned down for military service in World War 1 on medical grounds; it's unthinkable to contemplate that had it not been for this rejection, Bach might so easily have fallen with the millions of other victims of that conflict. We would never have inherited his legacy of the flower remedies! Bach spent the war years instead working at University College Hospital in his post of Assistant Bacteriologist. After the war he was appointed to the London Homeopathic Hospital. Homeopathic medicine was in those days, before the advent of antibiotics and the "superdrug" era, a much more accepted and mainstream form of medicine than it is now. It was at the Homeopathic Hospital that Bach first encountered, and became captivated by, the teachings of homeopathy's founder, Dr Samuel Hahnemann. Bach's early writings, before the development of the Bach flower remedies, included The Relation of Vaccine Therapy to Homeopathy (1920), Intestinal Toxaemia in its Relation to Cancer (1924), The Problem of Chronic Disease (1927), and The Rediscovery of Psora (1928).

From early on in his medical work, Bach was aware of the important role of the psychological and emotional outlook of his patients. He observed that those patients with a generally positive and optimistic outlook on life, who were able to remain cheerful even in their sick state, tended to respond better to treatment and make a better recovery from illness. Meanwhile, those patients with a more pessimistic, gloomy, bitter or depressive outlook on life, perhaps despairing of ever getting well again or being greatly affected by fear and anxiety about what was going to happen to them, tended to respond less well overall to treatment and were generally more prone to succumb to their illnesses. If they did recover, it was usually a much longer process.

Discovery of the mind-body connection

Dr Bach concluded from his observations that the emotions, psychological state, mindset and general attitude of a person must be a very significant factor in their overall state of wellbeing or constitutional strength. At the time his ideas were not taken seriously by the medical establishment, but in fact Bach had stumbled upon what is now an accepted concept in medicine, known by the rather long and unwieldy name of Psychoneuro-immunology (PNI for short). PNI is the study of how the state of mind can affect the state of physical health: for instance, the way a person suffering from chronic stress may have a lowered immune system and be prone to colds and viruses. Most doctors nowadays will readily accept the mind-body connection, as modern science has shown very conclusively that a poor state of mind will likely have an adverse effect on physical health sooner or later. Unhappy people become ill.

It's worth noting, however, that although the conventional medical scientific establishment now theoretically embraces this idea, in practice they have no real means of implementing it! Conventional therapies that act on the mind (mainly in the form of psychiatric drugs) can't have any significant PNI effect because they do not heal or cure psychological/emotional imbalances but instead simply bypass the symptoms by affecting brain chemistry. In general, once the drug treatment is stopped, the symptoms return within a short time showing that the root of the problem has not been touched. Almost a century after Dr Bach, our mainstream medical science is still cracking walnuts with sledgehammers and still unable to grasp the simple, subtle beauty of something like flower remedies.

Creation of the bowel remedies

In his bacteriological work Bach discovered further evidence to link the physical and mental/emotional states of his patients: broadly classing people into groups according to temperament, he noticed that there were correlations between their psychological type and the state of their bowel flora, i.e. the bacterial state of their gut and faeces. Anxious types of people tended to show up one particular bowel "picture"; angry types another, indecisive people another, and so on. On this basis, Bach created vaccinations derived from bowel flora and prescribed them largely according to patients' emotional states, with good results. However, Bach was dissatisfied. He was unhappy about working with the products of disease.

Discovery of homeopathy

Edward Bach's quest, from early on, was to find the most natural ways possible of relieving emotional suffering. When in 1919 he learned about homeopathy – at that time taken far more seriously by the conventional medical profession than it has been since the rise of the powerful pharmaceutical industry – he believed that he had discovered what he was looking for. He was attracted to homeopathy for its use of remedies that are nature-based, completely non-toxic and free of noxious chemical substances. He also approved of the fact that homeopathy's small innocuous remedies are mainly taken orally, as he disliked the idea of causing pain and injury to the patient by injecting them.

Bach attained fame as a homeopath when he created homeopathic versions from earlier bowel remedies: these were the Bowel Nosodes, derived from diseased human intestinal tissue and bowel flora but prepared homeopathically, extremely dilute and free from any noxious substances. The Bach Bowel Nosodes are still in use today as homeopathic remedies.

First plant remedies and discovery of the sunshine method

It was during his involvement with homeopathy that Dr Bach first experimented with making remedies from plants. These were homeopathic remedies, made by grinding (triturating) plant material and then subjecting it to the standard dilution/succussion homeopathic procedures to create different 'potencies' e.g. 30c, 200c, and so on. We know from his early writings, for instance, that his first version of the Impatiens remedy was 'triturated with sacc. lac. by hand... up to the seventh potency, after which succussion was adopted' (*Some New Remedies and New Uses*, published in *Homeopathic World*, February 1930).

Bach's homeopathic flower remedies were very effective at healing problems on both the physical and the mental/emotional levels: this early version of Impatiens, for example, was found effective in treating severe and acute pain as well as reducing accompanying fears and depression. Of course, this was nothing new to homeopathy, as a very large number of effective homeopathic remedies were already derived from flowers and plants.

Eventually, despite such successes, this highly idealistic doctor turned away from homeopathy altogether. He still wasn't satisfied, and wanted to find something that would come directly and unprocessed from nature, effective but completely gentle. And it wasn't long before he had found it. Sometime during 1930 he started using a very different and distinctly un-homeopathic system of making remedies. Instead of working in the laboratory as was – and still is – the practice in homeopathic pharmacy, Bach was now making his remedies out in the open air of the countryside.

His system was remarkably simple: he would place collected flower heads of a chosen type of flower into a glass bowl half-filled with ordinary water. The bowl containing water and flowers would be left to sit in the sun for two or more hours in a peaceful spot near where the flowers had been gathered. Then the water would be strained off, bottled and preserved with brandy. The flowers would be discarded. From these 'mother tincture' bottles, Bach would take two or three drops and place them in a second bottle, this time containing only neat brandy. From this bottle, containing the extremely dilute yet highly active flower-infused water, Bach would give a few drops at a time to patients suffering from emotional problems. Through extensive experimentation and trials he discovered that these new remedies were very effective and, just as importantly, completely safe.

The above method was known as the 'sunshine method'. Bach also employed a boiling method for making some of his remedies. With the boiling method, heat rather than sunlight was used to infuse the water with the qualities of the plant material. Afterwards, the water was strained off, the plant material thrown away, and from there the procedure was the same as the sunshine method of preparation.

Creation of the Bach flower remedies

In 1930 Bach closed his successful London medical practice, which had by then relocated to prestigious Harley Street. He felt that he had reached the end of his involvement with conventional medicine, as well as with homeopathy. He then packed his bags and set off on what he believed to be the completion of his life's mission, exchanging a stable and lucrative career for a life of uncertainty and increasing poverty to seek out the 'healing herbs' that would gently address the emotions and mental states of his patients. He was convinced that in setting up a new system that would ease the mind, he could create a radical new approach to addressing physical illness too.

In the last six years of his life – for he died at the young age of fifty – Bach focused all his attention on the creation of this new system of therapy. He threw himself into his work, seldom resting. He spent a great deal of time walking around the wild parts of England and Wales, gathering material from flowers, shrubs and trees, and continually experimenting. By 1936, the year he died, Bach had created a collection of thirty-seven flower remedies, one remedy that did not come from the plant kingdom but which was uniquely prepared from a source of water with reputed healing properties (Rock Water), and one further remedy which was a special combination of five of the flowers. Nowadays this five-in-one combination goes by various names depending on which company produces it – Five-Flower Formula, Recovery Remedy, Rescue Remedy.

From the 12 healers to the 7 categories

Those who read Dr Bach's original writings will be able to trace the progress of his developing collection. He started slowly and carefully, examining different plants and developing his methodology as he went along. Between September 1928 and the summer of 1932 he selected twelve plants and created remedies from them. These were: Agrimony/Cerato/Centaury/Chicory/ Clematis/Gentian/Impatiens/Mimulus/Rock Rose/Scleranthus/ Vervain/Water Violet. Excited by his discoveries, he first wrote about these remedies in his 1933 publication Twelve Healers, which you can still read today. As he added more remedies to his list, he kept revising his system in more books and articles. To his Twelve Healers he added four 'helpers', then expanded those four to seven, and so on. Dr Bach probably had no idea that he would finally collect as many as 38. The last nineteen remedies in his collection, often referred to as 'the Second Nineteen' were developed in rapid succession in a huge burst of inspired activity between March and July 1935 – contrast this to the first nineteen, which had taken him more than six years to develop.

Not long before he died, Bach experimented with a way to categorise his remedies. Perhaps, because there were now so many of them, he was thinking that he needed a way to group them together to help people choose which one they needed. Based on his observations of people and their emotions and behaviour, he came up with seven categories or headings:

1. **Fear**

2. **Uncertainty**

3. **Insufficient interest in present circumstances**

4. **Loneliness**

5. **Over-sensitivity to influences and ideas**

6. **Despondence and despair**

7. **Over-care for the welfare of others**

These categories are little used today. Many people find them confusing, and certainly, there are some problems with the system. For example, Dr Bach included his remedy Red Chestnut under **Fears**, when in fact it would have fitted much better under **Over-care for the welfare of others**. Red Chestnut helps when we are too worried about someone we love. Another example is the remedy Gorse, which can help with severe despair and feelings of hopelessness. Bach put this remedy under **Uncertainty** when it would have worked better under **Despondence and despair**, where (as we'll see later on) it would sit very well with remedies like Wild Rose. So while it's interesting to get an historical 'taste' of Dr Bach's original ideas, this experimental system of categories doesn't really work in practice. It works even less well for using Bach remedies with dogs or other animals, whose psychology is a little different from our own.

In this book, we won't attempt to categorise or group the remedies in any particular way, but will simply examine each one in turn, in the order in which Dr Bach discovered them. Later in the book we'll take a detailed tour of all 38 Bach flower remedies, looking at the properties and uses of each one in turn and how they apply to helping dogs. For the moment, below is a brief summary of the remedies as Dr Bach described them for helping human problems, giving a taste of what each one can be used for.

If you have never read about the Bach remedies before, note how many of the painful states of mind, negative attitudes and out of balance behavioural tendencies listed below are extremely commonplace in everyday life; and think what kind of a world we could have without them!

Overview of the Bach flower remedies

(Presented in chronological order of their discovery by Dr Bach)

1. *Impatiens:* Forcing one's own fast pace onto others; impatient, intolerant of people's mistakes or slowness to understand

2. *Mimulus*: Everyday fears of objects, people, circumstances; nervous anticipation of a coming event or situation

3. *Clematis*: Daydreaming, disconnected from the present moment, ungrounded, 'not with it'

4. *Agrimony*: Oversensitive to turmoil and quarrel; may seem outwardly cheerful but tormented by inner stress

5. *Chicory*: Self-centred and attention-seeking relationship to others, tends to bind others to them

6. *Vervain*: Overenthusiastic, over ideas or in general behaviour; hyper-energetic

7. *Centaury*: Wants to please and serve, but too open to the demands of others; neglecting own needs

8. *Cerato*: Inner uncertainty, lack of self-assurance, over-dependence on the advice of others

9. *Scleranthus*: Vacillation between options, delay in making decisions; tendency to hesitate and be unsure of oneself

10. *Water Violet:* Tendency to be too self-reliant to the point of shutting others out; closed off and hardened

11. *Gentian:* Discouragement that may come with setbacks and difficulties; urge to give up or not try anything new

12. *Rock Rose:* States of intense fear, terror and heightened nervousness

13. *Gorse:* Hopelessness, despair, gloomy attitude and retreat from active engagement in the world

14. *Oak:* States of stoic perseverance in the face of hardship and despair, leading to self-weakening and depletion of energy

15. *Heather:* Tendency to be fixated on oneself, one's problems, etc.; not wanting to talk of anything else

16. *Rock Water:* Tendency to be rigid, obsessive, stuck in a rut; too hard on oneself and trying to set an example

17. *Vine:* Tendency to be a bully, domineering, bossy, taking control of people or situations

18. *Olive:* Exhaustion and inability to attend to daily business

19. *Wild Oat:* Lack of motivation and incentive plus uncertainty in choosing a 'life path'

20. *Cherry Plum:* States of tension with fear of losing control of the rational mind: 'I'm going crazy'

21. *Elm:* Feeling overwhelmed and overburdened by tremendous tasks, unable to meet the challenge any more

22. *Aspen:* States of foreboding and vague haunting fears for which no explanation can be given

23. *Chestnut Bud:* Difficulty absorbing new ideas or retaining lessons; tendency to repeat the same error

24. *Larch:* Low self-esteem, lacking in confidence; sense that anything we try is doomed to failure

25. *Hornbeam:* Mental fatigue, listlessness, procrastination in the face of duties

26. *Willow:* Feeling not favoured by fate, or mistreated by others; developing bitterness and resentment

27. *Beech:* Tendency to be intolerant and critical of other people, with a judgmental outlook

28. *Crab Apple:* Unable to rise above 'shameful' aspects of the self and despairing over them

29. *Walnut:* Oversensitive and vulnerable to outside impressions, too affected by things

30. *Holly:* Easily upset and irritated by vexing and annoying circumstances; angry outlook

31. *Star of Bethlehem:* Burdens of grief, trauma and shock and their after-effects

32. *White Chestnut:* Mental agitation, pre-occupation or intense worry that seem to take over the whole mind and are hard to 'switch off'

33. *Red Chestnut:* Too bound up in worrying over the wellbeing of someone close; frustrated sense of helplessness

34. *Pine:* States of guilt and self-reproach, tendency to feel responsible or take on board blame for every little thing

35. *Honeysuckle:* Living in the past, belief that happiness can never be repeated again in the future

36. *Wild Rose:* Apathy and withdrawal, sense of giving up, wanting to retreat and fade away

37. *Mustard:* Withdrawal into depression and gloominess, lack of joy in life

38. *Sweet Chestnut:* Unbearable anguish and despair, deep emotional pain, sense of futility and joylessness

Between them, the Bach flower remedies cover an enormous range. Because they can be combined together, there are a virtually infinite number of possible ways they can work together to address the problems of any individual sufferer. This makes them a very individualised and personalised therapy, whether used to help a human or any other animal.

Tragically, Dr Bach was a very sick man in those last years while the flower remedies were being created. The cancer that had nearly killed him during his twenties had finally caught up with him again. It may be that Bach had burned himself out working so hard; or perhaps the reason he had worked so furiously to complete his system was that he knew he had limited time. We shall never know. When he died in November 1936 he was virtually penniless, having invested everything he had into his project. His only source of hope was his faith that his system of healing with flower remedies would bring relief to a suffering world.

It actually took many years for the Bach flower remedies to become widely known and used across the world. Bach's immediate followers, including Nora Weeks and Victor Bullen, kept up the Oxfordshire country house that had been Bach's base at the end of his life, and set up what is now the Edward Bach Foundation/Bach Centre. The production and promotion of the Bach flower remedies gradually grew into a successful business, reaching a high level of popularity from the 1970s and 80s onwards when there was a surge in public interest in complementary therapies. Eventually, the original business was sold to the homeopathic pharmaceutical company Nelsons for a large sum of money and a new division, Nelson Bach, was formed that has transformed the Bach flower business into a huge global industry. Meanwhile, other companies started producing their own versions of the Bach remedies. One such company is Ainsworths, also a homeopathic pharmacy. Another producer of Bach flower remedies is Healing Herbs Ltd, which has deliberately eschewed the mass-production path taken by the larger companies and adheres to the pure methods of Dr Bach, producing everything by hand and using only the purest, finest, organic ingredients. Many people believe that the final result of such an approach is a superior, more effective remedy.

Dr Bach's view of health and illness

Bach not only saw his remedies as important for helping with emotional problems, he also regarded them as very important in the context of medical treatment and physical health. This idea was based on his observations of sick patients: the happier and more cheerful patients tended to do better, while the unhappy or pessimistic, angry, despairing patients tended to be more vulnerable to their illness. In his Wallingford lecture, given on his 50th birthday shortly before he died, Bach outlined the four ways of using the remedies:

1. **Prevention of ill health**
   Keeping strong in mind/emotions by treating mental/emotional states as they arise. This can have a very powerful effect on our general immunity to illnesses, and our constitutional strength. Bach was one of the first doctors to

gain such an accurate insight into the medical importance of a positive mental attitude.

2. **Help stop illness at onset**
Dr Bach believed that by keeping the emotions bright and healthy, threatened illnesses could be prevented from developing; or at least, their effect could be reduced.

3. **Help during illness, once it has begun**
Dr Bach had seen the importance of helping sick patients regain and maintain their optimism and cheerfulness. He had noticed that happier people would respond better to treatment and recover more quickly from illness. It follows that using the Bach flower remedies can help the sick to recover more quickly, not by treating the direct cause of the illness but by supporting the patient's mental strength, optimism and resolve.

4. **Help with character traits that bring unhappiness**
Dispositions of character that cause problems for the sufferer can be gently transformed, allowing a happier and freer personality to emerge.

The Bach flower remedies: what they are, how they work

For many people, it's not important to understand how Bach remedies work, or even whether they've been 'proven' to work by scientists. Many of us are simply content to use them and see the benefits they offer to us, our loved ones and our companion animals. Indeed, there is a large and fast-growing body of anecdotal evidence to support the beliefs of millions of people that Bach flower remedies really do work as claimed. They are used across the world by many vets, doctors and other healthcare professionals who would have little interest in them if they weren't getting results! In Cuba, for instance, Bach remedies are now integrated into the national health system.

Nonetheless, like alternative and complementary therapy in general, Bach remedies are still an area of controversy. For all their millions of satisfied users, among the conventional medical establishment there is still much resistance to the idea that these odd little bottles can really contain anything worthwhile. Many readers of this book, who may never have seen a Bach remedy in action, may be hungry for more information that could persuade them to take this therapy seriously. So it would seem like a wasted opportunity merely to use this book to 'preach to the converted' and not to try to take a slightly deeper look for the benefit of readers who may be new to all this.

To the question 'do they work?' the answer is an emphatic yes, they do. The efficacy of Bach flower remedies is now well established through decades of reliable anecdotal evidence as well as a growing number of scientific studies (mainly on people). As to *how* they work, we'll come right out and say that nobody has ever demonstrated scientifically exactly, how Bach remedies are able to have the effect they do. However, there is enough peripheral scientific knowledge to be able to piece together a pretty good layperson's picture of what's going on inside the body when we take a Bach remedy or give one to a dog.

The tired old placebo argument

One of the arguments often 'trundled out' against Bach remedies is the claim that their apparent benefits are really nothing more than a placebo effect. This is a recognised effect whereby a person suffering from a given problem can be made better by giving them a 'placebo' remedy. A placebo remedy doesn't contain anything that might help – it might just be a little unmedicated sugar pill, or even just a glass of plain water – but works on the basis of the patient's trust and faith in their doctor and their belief that they will get better. And indeed, it's sometimes possible to 'trick' people into getting better this way. When drugs are being tested in medical trials, placebos are used as controls to show by comparison that the drug really works. Humans receiving placebo remedies usually show a 10% improvement on these 'blanks'. This is a fascinating insight into the power of the mind.

But is this the way Bach remedies work? The easiest way to argue against this theory is when we point out that Bach remedies help animals. You can't 'trick' an animal into getting better. In veterinary medical trials where drugs are being tested on animals, control groups are used to compare the progress of the animals given the drugs to those that are given nothing, but none of the animals given these 'blank' remedies show any placebo effect. With Bach remedies, the fact that a dog, cat, horse or bird can be helped is strong evidence that the Bach remedies really do work.

Bach remedies compared to other types of plant remedy

To get an understanding of how the Bach remedies work and what they really are, it's a good idea first of all to distinguish them clearly from other types of natural remedy that may at first sight seem very similar. Bach flower remedies are often confused with some of their cousins, other types of remedies derived from the plant kingdom, As we'll see, they're really very different indeed!

It's very easy to think of the Bach flower remedies as a type of herbal medicine. Another misconception is the confusion between flower remedies and essential oils. However, although they also come from plants, Bach flower remedies differ very greatly from either of these types of remedy.

Both herbal remedies and aromatherapy oils use the active biochemical properties of plants to bring about chemical changes to the body (affecting physical symptoms) and brain (affecting mental/emotional symptoms). Herbal remedies take the chemical properties of plants straight from nature, while essential oils are distilled and highly concentrated, and must generally be very well diluted. While these types of remedies aren't as powerful or as toxic as modern medical drugs, some care needs to be exercised in using them. Essential oils, for instance, must usually be heavily diluted before use, and users are advised to carry out 'patch tests' on small areas of skin before treatment, in case of irritation. It's also unsafe to give essential oils orally. Another problem with herbal remedies, that has recently been the subject of media discussion, is that some of them can interact with medical drugs – an example is St Johns Wort, which has been reported to contra-indicate, i.e. clash with, conventional anti-depressants such as Prozac.

However, although they also come from plants, Bach flower remedies differ very greatly from either of these types of remedy. They are 100% safe, they do not contain material doses of plant chemicals, and they can be used alongside any form of medication without any risk of adverse interactions. Completely unlike their herbal cousins, Bach flower remedies contain nothing of the chemical properties of the source plant. Spectroscopic analysis shows that Bach flower remedies are physically diluted to the point that they contain literally 'nothing' that can (using existing technologies) be measured or quantified, i.e. not one molecule of the source substance remains. This is why they have none of the perfume of an essential oil. They contain ONLY the water and the preservative that keeps the water in good condition (usually brandy). This means they are absolutely safe and non-toxic. It also could be taken to mean that they are absolutely useless! But practice shows them to be highly effective. How, then, do we explain how Bach remedies work?

Understanding energy

Bach flower remedies are what we call a dynamic therapy, as opposed to a material therapy that uses something tangible and measurable, to operate. e.g. chemicals. The Bach flowers use a particular form of subtle energy to work on our bodies and minds.

Living beings – including us and our dogs – are very much *energetic* in nature. What does this mean? No, it doesn't mean we're always jumping around and full of beans. It means that these fleshy bodies we inhabit are actually made of nothing more or less than energy. Every molecule of a living organism vibrates at a particular energetic (electromagnetic) frequency, and every living being has an unseen yet very real energy or bio-electrical field, which surrounds, penetrates and permeates the physical body. In fact, this energy field IS the physical body!

Sounds bizarre? Well, it sounded bizarre to physicists too, before Albert Einstein's physics revolution in 1905. Nowadays it's bread-and-butter knowledge that energy fields are actually more fundamental to reality than our normal concept of 'matter', and that visible matter is no more than a state of energy in varying stages of density. Physics shows, for example, that the chair you are sitting on to read this book is itself nothing more than a very dense conglomeration of energetic subatomic particles and that the interaction between it and your body – the fact that it supports you and you don't fall through it – is actually down to the interaction of the chair's and your body's respective electromagnetic fields.

For a practical understanding of this idea, try pressing two magnets together. You'll find they either attract or repel each other, depending on which poles you bring together. This repulsion is basically what keeps you from falling through the earth! Due to these same forces, when you turn this page, your fingers will not be physically touching the paper but rather it will be the energy field of your fingertips interacting with the energy field of the paper that enables you to move them. In other words, energy underlies and dictates all physical relationships between things, and is utterly crucial to the existence and stability of matter. What we sense with our five physical senses and feel with our emotional capacity is only the reflection, the by-product, of an unseen, supersensible realm of energy.

Scepticism and science

Modern biology is forced to follow where modern physics leads, and to a large extent it does. Unfortunately, one major corner of the biology world, the medical establishment, remains dominated by thinking that is now very outdated (by at least a century). It's this conventional thinking that puts up the big barriers to any form of energy therapy or medicine. It states that there must be molecules of a substance for that substance to have an effect. If there's 'nothing' in a remedy, according to this understanding it can't work and any reported effects must be due to placebo effect, i.e. a kind of faith healing. But we already know that the placebo effect can't account for the beneficial effects of Bach remedies on animals. Furthermore, where does this leave common medical technologies such as X-rays, ultrasound or lasers? There's 'nothing' in them either, yet they are well established at the heart of medical practice. Clearly, something else is going on.

Digital biology

Cutting-edge 'digital biology' sheds light on unanswered questions in science by revealing the nature of electromagnetic molecular signalling: that is, the way that information passes through the physical body. After eight years of research and in the course of thousands of replicated experiments, the late French scientist Dr Jacques Benveniste and his team at DigiBio Laboratories were able to transfer specific molecular energy signals onto a computer sound card. By playing these signals as sound (energy) waves to samples of material, they were able to lead receptor cells to 'believe' and act as though they were in the presence of the original molecules from which the signals had been gathered, even though they were not physically present.

In other words, one could say that biological systems function rather like radio sets, by a process of co-resonance. If you have a radio receiver tuned to a certain frequency, say BBC Radio 2, you will receive that signal from the transmitter vibrating at the same frequency. You won't find any molecules of Radio 2 in the miles of air between your radio and the broadcasting station! The wave that carries the information is a form of energy.

These are likely to be the kinds of activities going on in the body when we take a flower remedy, the sending of bio-resonant energy waves through tissue and water carrying digital healing information. According to this model, the Bach flower remedies operate by bio-electrical resonance.

Think of it as a subtle, hi-tech version of herbalism that dispenses with the crudeness of molecular chemistry. One could liken the difference to that between a mechanical instrument (akin to herbalism) and an electronic one (akin to Bach flower remedies). If herbs and essential oils are an abacus, Bach flower remedies are a high-performance computer.

Uploads and downloads

Bach flower remedies make use of the ability of simple water to retain or 'upload' the energy frequencies of a flower. When we take a Bach remedy, or give some to a dog, we are in a sense 'downloading' that information back into their system. The body's own energy system conducts the information in the form of very subtle energy waves which travel through water and tissue. The energy field of the flower, carried in the water, is able to interact with the field of the recipient and influence its state. This effect then filters down, by a complex process of electrochemical conversions, into the conscious mind as improved mental/emotional/psychological wellbeing.

Each different type of flower has a slightly different energy and carries slightly different 'information' into our system. This means that each of the 38 Bach remedies is able to address and influence a slightly different aspect of our energy field. But what they all have in common is that they are capable of healing blockages and imbalances at the highest and most subtle level of our being and that of animals. This highest level is the realm of the mind and emotions, the psychological state – or, if we dare to risk using such terms, the 'heart and soul'.

Bach remedies in the future

In distant years to come, we may find flower remedy therapy entering a complete new phase of scientific development. It may even one day be possible to convert the energy forms of Bach flower remedies into sound waves, permitting us to play them through speakers, or even construct 'scanners' that patients could simply walk through to receive the healing benefits. Once converted to a digital medium that our computers could read, we could download flower remedies from the Internet, carry them around on recording media such as CDs, and email them to each other! At present, the state of the art remains the highly effective and perfectly practical liquid format originally devised by Dr Edward Bach.

Chapter Two

Bach Flower Remedies
and Dogs

Helping animals, including dogs, has always been a part of the scope of Bach flower therapy. From the early days, Dr Bach saw that his remedies would benefit not just humans but all living creatures, even ailing plants. However, Bach's central interest was in helping people, not animals, and there was very little work or research carried out on the ways that the remedies could address animal problems. The Bach Centre in England has archives dating back to the 1950s that document some successful cases of the flower remedies being used in animal care. But it has only been in recent years that there has been a concentration of interest in the application of Bach flower remedies for animals.

The changing attitude towards animals and their emotional lives

It seems obvious to many animal carers that something like the Bach remedies, able to help with emotional and psychological problems, could have a vitally important role to play in animal care. But it's taken a very long time for a new, modern approach to animal care to start to emerge that addresses the emotional and psychological needs of animals in a more modern and intelligent way.

Why did it take so long for this to gather momentum and interest? We have to remember that attitudes have come a long, long way during the course of the last century. In Edward Bach's time, the majority of domestic animals were still very much part of industry. The famous James Herriot novels, describing the life of a vet in 1930s rural England, give interesting insights into attitudes to animals at that period in history. People's attitudes to animals were very utilitarian and, by definition, old-fashioned. Especially in country areas, animals were regarded primarily as either a source of food or materials, a means of transport or a tool of agriculture. Horses were mainly used for pulling carts, barges and ploughs, and the purpose of the dog was almost solely as a sheepdog, hunting dog or guard dog. Even though people did of course form close bonds with their dogs, it was something of a novelty to keep one 'only' as a pet or companion, and in fact many vets were opposed to the idea. The concept of a dog as a fully sentient and psychologically complex being capable of an enormous range of emotions, just like humans, would have been considered quite radical and probably rather odd.

So the emergence of a natural therapy that addresses the emotional needs of animals and recognises their great psychological complexity had to wait for more modern, more enlightened times.

Are we there yet? Almost! The 'old order' is always stubbornly resistant to change. Orthodox science has until very recently held that all animal behaviour could be attributed to pure "hard-wired" instinct – and is still, after all these years, echoing the traditional view that has prevailed since the time of the early scientist Descartes (who held that animals could not reason and therefore could not feel pain). Only in very recent times have new studies and new attitudes slowly begun to overturn traditional views of animals and to confirm what animal lovers and the more progressive animal behaviourists have known for many years: namely that animals share with humans the capacity for psychological suffering and problems such as depression, grief, heartbreak, confusion, loneliness, even loss of the will to live under certain circumstances. Today, we stand on the brink of a new era where the intelligence, emotional sophistication and sensitivity of animals as sentient beings will be properly and widely understood.

Dogs are not the only ones benefiting from our newfound wisdom. Studies carried out at Purdue University in the United States have demonstrated that pigs kept in isolation pens and deprived of contact with other pigs are liable to depression, with – as Dr Bach would have been able to tell them early last century! – a negative effect on their general health. In response to the study and as part of a new spirit of change in attitudes on animal rights, the European Union has outlawed the use of isolation pig pens by the year 2012. After this time, these social and intelligent animals will be required by law to be kept in open-air stalls where they can have contact with each other. Other studies, for instance on elephants in the wild, have demonstrated the capacity of animals to feel grief at the death of a companion. The biologist Joyce Poole has written that elephants' behaviour with the dead bodies of fellow herd members "leaves me with little doubt that they experience deep emotion and have some understanding of death".

In a move that will ultimately shake one of the great pillars of human culture to its roots – i.e. the belief in human superiority over the animal kingdom – we are realising that animals have a far greater sense of Self than we previously gave them credit for. The pioneering work of Dr Irene Pepperberg, with the now-famous African Grey parrot Alex, has produced findings that many people find rather hard to digest. An animal that we used to think was a "bird brain" is actually turning out to be quite the opposite! Alex has been able to master tasks that were long thought to be the exclusive domain of humans, notably the rational use of language. When learning to identify and name, in English, a variety of different colours, Alex saw himself reflected in a mirror. Peering at his reflection, he asked his handler "what colour am I?". The handler responded: "you are grey". After that, Alex was consistently able to identify and name the colour grey. Dr Pepperberg, a respected University Professor of Psychology and certainly no quack, has stated her belief that Alex will one day be able to read. Koko the gorilla, famous for learning sign language and understanding several thousand English words, has consistently scored between 70 and 95 in human IQ tests (placing her in the slow learner, but not retarded, category).

New attitudes to animal emotional and cognitive capabilities have begun to pave the way for a potential revolution in the way we regard and treat our fellow creatures, and these philosophical considerations have begun to trickle into courtrooms around the world as we are forced to review the future of our co-relationship with this planet's non-human inhabitants. Germany recently became the first country in the world to guarantee animal rights under its constitution. Human nature being what it is, when it comes to singling out species for animal rights reviews, we tend to favour those with the highest DNA similarity to humans, i.e. the apes! Evidently, we find it difficult to let go of our anthropocentric – human-centred – attitude.

But there's no doubt that, slowly but surely, our attitudes are changing. As well as setting the scene for important legal changes, these rapidly evolving attitudes towards animals' degree of sophistication and emotional sensitivities are accelerating the development of advanced and compassionate healthcare. The growth of interest in using therapies such as Bach flower remedies to help animals is the marriage of modern, progressive ideas about our fellow creatures combined with the use of a high-tech, ultra-sophisticated science of nature that is rapidly becoming verifiable in the light of modern physics and biology. In short, Bach flower therapy is destined to become a major part of the future of animal care as we move into a more enlightened age. And that is very exciting.

Helping people and dogs with Bach remedies

Helping dogs with Bach remedies is much, much more satisfying than helping humans! As any psychologist will tell you, humans can be tough to help. Sometimes they don't really want to be helped – they often resist getting better as they secretly or unconsciously relish the attention they get when they're depressed or miserable; other times, people are unwilling to let go of an emotional "crutch" that they've latched on to for support, such as alcohol or drugs, eating disorders or other types of behaviour. Humans with repressed emotional lives often recoil from confronting issues in their lives that they'd simply prefer not to think about – these can be things about themselves that they don't want to deal with, or aspects of their lives that are too frightening or painful to face up to. It's often easier for humans simply to go on repressing their pain, or redirecting their neuroses in ways that give them solace even though they may be harmful. So when humans are faced with a therapy like Bach flower remedies that offer them the potential for freedom from all these problems, which can start the process of loosening the knots that have gained a stranglehold on their personality, they may sometimes shy away. These emotional problems are often disguised as scepticism: it's easier to say 'I don't believe in that stuff' than it is to admit 'I'm terrified of throwing my crutch away'.

When it comes to helping an animal such as a dog, we can breathe a big sigh of relief, because animals present no such difficulties. Dogs are psychologically far healthier than most of us humans. Their concept of social values comes from their ancestor the wild wolf. If humans all disappeared tomorrow, dogs would simply return to their ancient wolf society. Wolf societies, called packs, are well organised, efficient, and free from cruelty. They never go to war, never harm one another without cause. They honour members of their own social groups and selflessly work for the collective benefit of their pack. They don't hold false ideas and delusions, don't suffer from pride and hate, and have no sense of greed and envy. How wonderful it would be if human societies could be as peaceful and harmonious as the world of the wolf and its descendant the dog! The authors have often speculated that the ancient philosophical art of Zen, whose goal is to liberate humans from the wants and desires of their ego, has already been attained by animals and in this respect they may be morally and spiritually superior to humans!

Perhaps because they're so much closer to nature already, and have such a "head start" on us, they often tend to respond faster and better to the remedies than humans do. A dog's recovery from emotional stress or psychological pain is a much simpler and uncomplicated business, and anyone who's ever helped a dog with Bach remedies can testify to the great satisfaction it brings to watch them changing, softening, losing their fear, regaining trust, learning to leave behind a difficult past, reclaiming their natural state of contentedness and vitality. You never lose the sense of wonder that comes with being able to help alleviate a dog's, or any animal's, emotional suffering with flower remedies.

Key areas for canine Bach flower therapy

There are several basic key areas of Bach flower therapy for dogs and other animals. These are typical types of negative emotional/ psychological states, situations or problems that seem to come up again and again and are the basis for much of canine Bach therapy.

Effects of past trauma

One of the most important areas of animal flower therapy is helping dogs who have been adversely and lastingly affected by psychological (or for that matter physical, insofar as it may involve great fear) traumatic experiences. Examples of what can constitute a past trauma include:

- Experienced acute moments of fear, terror, pain, beatings, attacks from people or other animals.

- Chronic situations the dog has had to endure, such as periods of ongoing cruelty from previous owners, daily extreme stress from being ill treated, starved or confined, living with very neurotic owners or in dysfunctional, unhappy or violent homes.

- Any kind of accident, shock, period of stress or other unpleasant incident.

Any dog that has been exposed to these kinds of stimuli for any length of time can be seriously affected and suffer terrible ongoing mental stress as a result. Animal rescue workers, who deal daily with cruelty cases and animals that have been psychologically abused, are all too aware of the suffering caused to their charges, and the tendency for a badly frightened, traumatised animal to fall physically ill, in just the same way as an emotionally traumatised human being can decline into poor health. Even with medical care and a good diet, many of these animals remain unhealthy until their fears, stress and past traumas are helped. Bach flower remedies are an ideal way of helping to achieve this. What the Bach flower remedies, notably Star of Bethlehem, are uniquely able to do is to target the underlying traumatic experience, the cause of the problem, even if it happened a long time previously. The remedies can also be used to address the problems that have been created by the traumatic experience, which are the symptoms we see in the dog's behaviour telling us that all isn't well. These can be things such as fear, nervousness, lack of confidence, dislike of men, and so on.

Fears and anxiety

Fear or anxiety, in its various forms, is one of the biggest problems suffered by dogs. The physiological symptoms of fear in a dog are so similar to those of a human being that it's highly realistic to assume the dog is experiencing this emotional state in much the way we do, and so it's very important to try to help them with this distressing state. Fear is easy to spot in a dog by observing certain tell-tale symptoms:

- Body carriage: The tail may be held between the legs, the dog's body carriage will be low, he will keep his head down and have a nervous expression on his face. When called, a nervous dog will tend to take a curved approach rather than walk up to you in a straight line.

- Submissive posture: The dog may roll over in submission at the slightest provocation, or urinate out of fear.

- Escape from perceived threat: Dogs that are fearful will often run and hide in whatever place they think is safe.

- Fearful aggression: Many dogs become fearfully aggressive as a result of bad experiences (see Effects of Past Trauma, above). This is just the dog's way of trying to protect himself against a perceived threat. Sometimes a dog may growl and then cringe, showing that he's really afraid of asserting himself, and thinks he's bound to be punished. Rescued dogs or dogs that have previously lived in homes where they may have been punished or beaten, often have this kind of mixture of aggressive and fearful behaviour.

More everyday examples of fear and anxiety are fear of travelling, fear of loud noises, fear of certain people, places, objects or situations. Bach flower remedies have a major role to play in helping to reduce this enormous problem.

Stress

Care and prevention of stress reactions is another important area in animal Bach flower therapy. Although their emotional lives may not be as complex as ours in some ways, they are just as capable of becoming stressed, anxious, confused, depressed and insecure. Managing stress levels for all animals will help to keep their immune system in good shape and help prevent the onset of illness – or if it does strike, it can help their systems to deal with it more efficiently. Canine stress can show up in a number of ways:

- Restless behaviour: The dog may chase his tail, pace up and down or round and round, and never seem to relax.

- Scratching and fur pulling: As a way to try to compensate for the stress, dogs can develop various 'redirected behaviours' including fur-pulling and chewing. They may lick a paw or leg until the skin is damaged and they have chronic wounds called lick granulomas. This is often simply due to long-term stress that has been unrecognised and untreated.

- Tension in muscles: The whole body may feel stiff and the dog's gait can be awkward. Stiffness like this can result from a state of prolonged mental stress. When the stress and mental tension is eased, there can be a relaxing of the physical level soon afterwards.

- Dog seems to be depressed: A depressed dog will tend to have little energy and spend a lot of time lying around. He might have a dull look about him, as though he has lost his 'vital spark'. Always check with the vet to make sure nothing is physically wrong with the dog. It's often the case that such a dog will have nothing wrong with him physically/medically, but just feels emotionally low and depressed.

- Excessive barking: Excessive barking is often the reason why dogs end up in the dog rescue system, because owners can't cope with the barking and get rid of the dog. Some owners will just abandon the dog. Excessive barking can sometimes be an attention-seeking type of behaviour, and it often happens with dogs suffering from separation anxiety, left alone all day. Other stressed dogs can bark all the time. Interestingly, there have been cases when wolves started barking after being taken into captivity. Wolves do not normally bark. The bark, which we always think of as a normal dog sound, may actually be an expression of stress. Many owners of happy, unstressed dogs report that they hardly ever, or never, hear their dogs barking.

- Excessive panting, when not thirsty: Normal panting comes when a dog is thirsty or after exercise. But a dog suffering from stress may pant at other times, perhaps even all the time.

- Destructiveness in the home: Stressed dogs may try to escape from their 'prison' by digging through doors or even walls. They may redirect their stress by chewing things to pieces. They may, in really bad cases, even chew themselves.

- Tendency to suffer from allergies: Dogs that have suffered a lot of stress over a long period can suffer a weakening of their immune system and be prone to allergies. If your dog has allergies it doesn't necessarily mean he's suffering from stress, but this is one possible factor.

- Poor coat condition: Patchy, matted, dry, shedding coats, or coats that lack lustre and vitality, may be signs of stress. They could also be signs of physical illness, so always check this isn't the case.

- Digestive or bowel problems: Just like humans, there are cases where certain dogs (often those rescued from shelters) suffer from long-term stomach problems, e.g. colitis, due to past or present stress. Using Bach remedies is an important part of solving these problems, although, because the stress has now had this chronic physical effect, it may be necessary to use other therapies also. Homeopathy and magnet therapy have been known to help with these problems.

Physical stress-related conditions

The question of treating stress-related or emotional problems that have had an effect on the physical body is a complex issue. Dr Bach claimed in his writings that treating the mental/emotional problem behind the physical illness was enough to cure the physical illness. This was what he meant when he said we should 'treat the person, not the disease'.

Was Dr Bach right about this? In lighter cases, when stress is causing minor physical problems that have not been there for very long, there's no doubt that Bach remedies can have a very good indirect effect on the physical level. However, in more serious cases, such as chronic stomach ulcers that have their roots in stress, Bach remedies can heal the mental/emotional or stress often not been shown to cure the s that suffer prolonged or extreme at may have been beaten or suffered go on to suffer immune system sical disease, can benefit from Bach nal and behavioural problems, but ed on to treat the physical illnesses . Nonetheless, the Bach remedies ementary part of the dog's overall

h therapy for dogs:

m the fact that dogs can soak up egativity of the people they live with. Certain flower remedies, notably Bach's Walnut, have the ability to offer protection against negative atmospheres by reducing the dog's sensitivity to them. The negative influences that most affect dogs are the emotional energies projected by unhappy or angry, bitter people – that atmosphere you can "cut with a knife" that lingers in the homes of argumentative families and people suffering from prolonged stress. Flower remedies can be extremely useful to help the people too, for their own sake and for the sake of the dogs who have to live with them!

Training and cognitive skills enhancement

Flower remedies are also useful in helping to socialise, teach and train dogs of all ages: from young and exuberant dogs that are bursting with energy and tending to run off in all directions, to older dogs that are set in their ways and tending not to absorb lessons. Bach flower remedies can help overcome different problems and barriers in the learning and training process, and we will be exploring this in more detail as we go on.

Recuperation from illness

This is another major area for this therapy. Whether an animal is receiving conventional medication, homeopathy or some other therapy, Bach flower therapy is of great benefit as an adjunct therapy helping the animal to cope and maintain vital energy through what may be a long haul. In many cases, flower remedies have been used as a "pick me up" for animals that risked not recovering after an operation when their vital energy has dipped very low. Older dogs are especially prone to long-drawn out recoveries from illness, and the psychological boost offered by certain Bach remedies can be extremely important to help them back on their feet. One of the real virtues of these remedies is that they can be given alongside any type of medication, and so are ideally suited to playing a complementary role for sick or recuperating animals.

Pet bereavement

This is another important area of use for the Bach remedies, and later in the book we devote a section to it to see how they can be used to help. Humans and dogs are equally affected by the death of a companion. Many dogs will go into a state of deep depression after losing a friend (either an owner or another dog). As for us, most people who have had dogs are all too familiar with the sense of loss when one dies. Certain Bach remedies are very important in helping ease the pain of pet loss.

Helping people and animals together

Helping the animals themselves is only a part of the picture. Wild animals have the freedom of being truly independent from us, and free to get on with their lives as nature intended. The lives of domesticated animals, however, are very bound up with those of the humans who live with them, care for them and attend to their needs. For these animals, life is rather more complex and fraught with potential problems, many of them the direct or indirect result of being in partnership with this strange two-legged species we call Homo Sapiens. This partnership needs to be regarded as a whole to really understand its dynamics and how to solve any problems that might arise within it. Animal problems and human problems are very often two sides of the same coin, and Bach flower remedies can be used to promote greater harmony for all, enriching our relationships with animals and theirs with us.

When Bach remedies might not be the best or only approach

It's important to realise that many canine behavioural problems may have a variety of causes. If, for instance, a dog has become aggressive or depressed, it may be a mistake to judge this purely as an emotional or psychological problem – he could be in pain, or be suffering from some other medical disorder whose treatment lies outside the jurisdiction, or effective range, of Bach flower therapy. So, when faced with a situation where a dog is acting or behaving in a way that we think he needs help, what steps can we take to decide whether this is a 'Bach flower case' or not?

- First make absolutely sure that there's nothing medically wrong with the dog that could be distressing him, by checking with the vet. Flower remedies can help to alleviate mental stress associated with pain or illness, but aren't the appropriate treatment for the pain or illness itself. If it turns out that the dog is ill or in pain, we can use Bach remedies to help together with what the vet does.

- Second, it could be at least partly a training issue. Perhaps the dog is spoilt? Perhaps the owner (or previous owner) has accidentally taught the dog that certain behaviours are acceptable. Perhaps the dog feels he has every right to growl at you when you try to handle him or make him get off your armchair or bed. This sort of behaviour occurs very often when owners allow this very hierarchy-conscious animal to get the idea that he's as high up in the pack order as they are. It can actually cause a great deal of stress to a dog to let him rise to a leadership position within the pack, letting him have access to all areas, letting him take charge of all situations, deciding when to start or end a play session, and so on. Some dogs are temperamentally suited as individuals to be the leader, while for others it would be like giving a super-high-stress executive job to someone who isn't able to deal with the load. Many canine behaviour problems start this way. To reverse this trend is more of a training issue than a call for flower remedies. Flower remedies can help with re-training a poorly trained dog, but will not in every case bring about a satisfactory cure all on their own. This is because if you have given your dog the impression that it's OK to growl at visitors or bite the cat, he isn't suffering an emotional imbalance by doing so, but merely behaving like a dog! In such a case, flower remedies should be used in a complementary role to some appropriate behaviour work, perhaps guided by a canine behaviourist. There's also a lot that the owner can do at home to help the dog to re-learn more appropriate behaviours. See *Resources* at the end of the book for more information.

Other important considerations

Here are some more points to take into account when considering what kind of help a dog needs from you:

1. *Is your dog getting enough exercise?* All dogs, but certain breeds in particular such as border collies, which were bred to burn up a great deal of energy, can become stressed and unhappy if not given enough exercise.

2. *Is he on a good healthy diet?* Poor or inappropriate feeding can cause behavioural problems such as hyperactivity. There have been cases where Bach remedies only had a partial effect because the real cause of the problem was dietary. There are some very high-quality canine diets commercially available, such as Burns, James Wellbeloved and NatureDiet (see *Resources* at the end of the book). Sometimes only trial and error will tell what diet an individual dog thrives on best. If in doubt, check with your vet.

3. *Does he get enough mental stimulation?* Dogs are intelligent, social animals that will become bored and depressed if starved of social interaction, play and fun activities, and a sense of companionship.

4. *Or too much?* Overstimulation, such as too many games leading to lack of rest, can be stressful. This is especially true of young pups, which need a lot of rest.

5. *Has he got a safe place of his own?* Every dog should have his own space where he can retreat and feel secure. Even a simple plastic dog bed in a corner, with an old duvet laid inside for comfort, will provide the security of a cosy den.

6. *Is he picking up on your negative emotions?* Bach remedies alone will never entirely protect a dog from stress in the home if there's an unhappy atmosphere or constant arguments going on. We owe it to our dogs, as well as to ourselves, to try to lead happier and more relaxing daily lives.

7. *Has he lost a companion recently, or have there been any other changes in circumstances?* Always think carefully what might have triggered a behavioural or emotional problem in a dog. By identifying the exact cause of the problem – for instance perhaps the dog's best friend, an older dog, just died; or perhaps you recently moved to a different home – helps to pick out the Bach remedy or remedies that will be most effective in helping relieve the problem.

Chapter Three

The 38 Remedies

In this main section of the book we're going to take a guided tour of the whole collection of remedies created by Dr Bach. To help gain an authentic historical flavour of Bach's work, the remedies are examined in the order he developed them.

Each remedy is examined from a human, and then a canine perspective. This not only allows us to develop a closer feeling for the use of each remedy, it also gives interesting insights into some of the similarities and differences in the ways that humans and dogs think, feel and perceive the world about them. It's always important to bear in mind that many of the emotional and psychological states that occur in humans are not found in dogs, or are experienced and expressed in a different way by the dog. One of the dangers of interpreting the uses of Bach remedies for dogs is to fall into the trap of anthropomorphic thinking, that is, to ascribe human characteristics to animals. Dogs are actually very lucky that they aren't as crazy as humans! This means that, although each and every Bach remedy has a potential use within canine care, some of the Bach flower remedies are less frequently used for animals than for people. In this section, Bach remedies that are found to be the most often needed and used for dogs (and other animals) are marked with an asterisk (*).

Although we'll be looking at the remedies individually, the reader should be aware from the start that the best results with this therapy are often obtained when using remedies in combination with one another. It's possible to combine up to 8 or so Bach remedies, addressing different elements or 'angles' of a problem. We'll be learning more about this later in the book. In the meantime, a good knowledge of each individual remedy will help you to create effective combinations later on.

IMPATIENS*

Latin name:	Impatiens glandulifera
Dr Bach's words:	'Those who are quick in thought and action and wish all things to be done without hesitation and delay. When ill they are anxious for a hasty recovery'
Keynotes:	**Impatience, frustration, pressure, stress**
Goal of therapy:	**To restore a sense of relaxation and serenity**

Impatiens for People: The very first remedy Dr Bach developed is also one of the most important. Impatiens is a remedy for an impatient, pressing, driving state of mind: a state of tension. The mind is wound-up, with a sense of urgency to move fast and 'get things done'. Such people may regard themselves as the leader in any situation – and in fact quite often the Impatiens 'type' of person is very capable and quick-thinking. The remedy is needed when natural skill and leadership tend to border over into ruthlessness, intolerance, anger, frustration, dissatisfaction and irritability – all of which take their toll and make it hard for the person to gain inner peace. The state doesn't switch off when the person is off-duty, either, but stays in the mind, gnawing away constantly. The goal of the remedy is to help give inner peace and freedom from restless pressure and agitation.

Impatiens for Dogs: If we think about it, the use of Impatiens basically boils down to how we respond to, and deal with, stress. Dogs by nature are very patient animals, and they don't normally need a remedy like Impatiens to help with impatient or demanding character traits of this kind as a human might. However, the key thing here is the ability of the Impatiens remedy to help relax the mind and reduce stress and, as dogs are very susceptible to mental stress, it's in this way that the remedy can help them most.

Any situation where a dog seems over-wrought, tense, worried, stressed, can call for the Impatiens remedy to bring greater calm. For instance, it could be used to help soothe the mind of a dog that is recovering from illness or undergoing medical treatment, when he may feel irritable, restless and generally uptight. If a dog seems to have a 'highly-strung' temperament, Impatiens is one remedy that could be used to help reduce stress or tension levels. (It would be wise to check with a vet that this state of tension, if it's an ongoing thing, doesn't indicate some kind of medical issue such as a nagging pain or other source of discomfort. It's also important, if a dog seems continually stressed, to try to identify what might be causing it. Later in the book we examine some of the ways that humans can inadvertently cause stress to their dogs inside or outside the home.)

Impatiens is a component of the famous Bach combination remedy, variously known as Five-Flower Formula, Recovery Remedy or Rescue Remedy, and it's probably in this role that the remedy is most often given to dogs. The classic combination of Impatiens/Rock Rose/Cherry Plum/Clematis and Star of Beth-lehem is a very useful remedy indeed to have to hand in case of any upsetting, shocking, stressful incident that could befall either a dog, his owner, or both.

MIMULUS*

Latin Name:	Mimulus Guttatus
Dr Bach's words:	'Fear of accidents, of unknown things, of people, of strangers, of crowds, of being alone, of the dark... the fears of everyday life'
Keynotes:	**General fears and anxiety, nervousness**
Goal of therapy:	**To restore confidence and calm**

Mimulus for People: The Mimulus remedy is for all those everyday fears, such as being anxious in regard to something concrete – for humans this includes things like a driving test or an exam, or having to stand up in public and give a talk. Generally, Mimulus is indicated for anticipated fearful events, fears of known objects, people or situations. People chronically in need of Mimulus are often shy and retiring, may not openly share or express their fears, but are generally nervy and fearful and tend to lack a strong character.

Mimulus for Dogs: The remedy is used in much the same way for dogs as for people. Dogs needing Mimulus will tend to be underconfident and have fears of certain things, perhaps situations where they feel scared and vulnerable. The positive effect of Mimulus on dogs is to encourage greater confidence and help them to deal with situations better.

Mimulus is a very commonly used remedy for dogs, as many of their problems are related to fear, anxiety and nervousness. Fear of a more acute or extreme type, which could be described as a state of terror, calls for a different Bach remedy, Rock Rose. This can be given in addition to Mimulus, or perhaps simply instead of it. Mimulus may help with quite severe fears in dogs, but tends to work more slowly than Rock Rose, because it's dealing with less extreme, less sudden and less acute states of fear and anxiety.

Research has shown that a fear remedy like Mimulus tends to address the outer 'layer' of the dog's mental state, and while it can be very useful in helping with fears, if the fear stems from something like a past trauma (this could be anything from an attack by another dog to a car accident, to an experience of cruel treatment in the past) you may find that best results will be obtained from combining the fear remedy with another that will act on the root of the trauma. For this, see Star of Bethlehem.

CLEMATIS*

Latin name:	Clematis vitalba
Dr Bach's words:	'Those who are dreamy, drowsy, not fully awake, not really happy in their present circumstances... in illness some make little or no effort to get well'
Keynotes:	**Indifference, boredom, detachment**
Goal of therapy:	**To restore focus, interest and concentration**

Clematis for People: Discovered not very long after Impatiens, Bach's Clematis is really the complete antithesis of the earlier remedy. While Impatiens helped with impatient, pressing states of mind, Clematis is a remedy that helps the opposite state, that of dreaminess and a sense of not being 'with it'. People needing Clematis are not fully grounded in the here and now. They are somehow detached, dreamy, disconnected, and may seem very distracted when you are talking to them. Sometimes they may long for better times, life in the present appears boring and unfulfilling. They may spend much time daydreaming, and suffer from sleepiness and a lack of mental alertness. The remedy helps to restore these, and also to help in stressful situations where people react by becoming slow-thinking and 'out of it'. This is the reason Clematis was included in the famous 'Rescue Remedy' emergency formula.

Clematis for Dogs: We don't really know a great deal about what goes on in the inner mind of a dog. It would be easy to state that dogs don't have romantic longings or spend time dreaming about fantasies. However, some dogs are observed to seem to live 'in their own world', as though disconnected from things around them – so who knows what thoughts might be going through their minds? That dogs dream is well established: they are often seen to 'run' in their sleep, make little sounds that indicate they are somewhere far away in their imagination, and even have the occasional nightmare just like us. It's not unfeasible that dogs don't share with us the ability to daydream from time to time, and maybe some of them, like us, are more prone to it than others! The authors' Cavalier spaniel, Pagan, is one such dog who seems to slip into a little world of her own, a contented state of dreaminess.

Most of the time, this isn't a problem – and we, for one, are happy to let little Pagan enjoy whatever dreamy inner world she is visiting. However there may be times when it would benefit the dog to gently restore a bit more mental focus: if, for instance, the dreamy state is suspected of being the dog's withdrawal into himself as a way of coping with stress. In such a case, Clematis would be good to team up with a remedy like Impatiens, as well as another we haven't looked at yet, Wild Rose. If the dreamy state were possibly connected to a past trauma of some kind – for instance if a dog from a rescue shelter with an unknown past tended to withdraw a lot into himself, you might think of combining Clematis, Wild Rose and Star of Bethlehem.

Clematis also has a use in helping to train dogs. Training dogs is really just about helping them to learn new ideas and associations. This requires mental focus, and just like a child who doesn't seem to concentrate, a dreamy or disconnected dog will tend not to learn very much. Clematis can work well here together with the Bach remedy Chestnut Bud, which has a key use in helping the dog to retain the lessons of training.

AGRIMONY*

Latin Name:	Agrimonia eupatoria
Dr Bach's words:	'People who love peace and are distressed by argument or quarrel, to avoid which they will agree to give up much'
Keynotes:	**Mental torture and worry, sensitivity to disturbances and disharmony**
Goal of therapy:	**To restore inner peace and tranquillity**

Agrimony for People: Agrimony is a remedy that helps people who are very easily subjected to worries, discord, or commotion. They carry a burden of anxiety that becomes too much to bear if weighted by any additional pressure from the outside. However, rather than try to deal with the anxiety that is gnawing at them, they often endeavour to hide or suppress it behind a veneer of false cheerfulness. This sometimes leads to a varying degree of dependence on alcohol or drugs. The kind of person who surprises all their friends and family by falling into a deep and sudden depression after years of seeming cheerful and happy, is a classic 'Agrimony type'. What the remedy does is to help free the mind from that inner pressure of anxiety. Sometimes trapped unconscious feelings are brought to the surface before being released. The person may go through a brief phase where one comes face-to-face with these upsetting emotions, but this temporary so-called 'healing crisis' should not be regarded as a negative thing but rather a cathartic and healthy experience.

Agrimony for Dogs: Dogs are very peace-loving creatures. Their natural social groups are designed to avoid conflict and to live in harmony together, and in their natural state they would suffer none of the psychological stress of living in a dysfunctional environment. Unfortunately, because we have brought this animal into the unnatural and problematic human world, they are often compelled to live with people who are unhappy and shout and argue with one another. Dogs are very affected if they have to live in an atmosphere of conflict or quarrel. They would do almost anything to make this stop, though they have no power to make this happen. They will wait patiently for it to be over, trying to keep out of the way and feeling very stressed. If this situation happens often, it will become a source of chronic stress for the dog. The dog may become nervous and confused, or even quite depressed. Dogs that suffer from this kind of stress can be helped with Agrimony, but it's also important for people to address their own emotional problems.

Agrimony can help any dog suffering from stress, and as such it makes a good companion to the Bach remedy Impatiens. Another related remedy is Walnut, helping dogs to deal with stressful outside influences. These three remedies in combination can be very helpful to ease the stress of situations like kenneling, confinement at the vet's, quarantine, introduction to a new pack or any other experience that could be disquieting to them.

Some writers have described the 'Agrimony dog' as a dog that hides his tension and unhappiness from people and 'tries to please' or act falsely cheerful even though he's very stressed and mentally tortured. This is failing to understand the way dogs think, and in practice this simply doesn't happen. If a dog is stressed and unhappy, he will show it! There is absolutely no reason why a dog would try to pretend otherwise, and as far as we know there is no evidence that a dog has ever done this.

Another important difference between humans and animals is highlighted by the Agrimony remedy. This is the fact that, when helped with an emotional problem such as chronic stress, a dog or other animal can't suffer any sort of 'healing crisis' as part of the therapy. Luckily for dogs, their response to Bach remedies is straightforward, positive and uncomplicated.

CHICORY*

Latin name:	Cichorium intybus
Dr Bach's words:	'Those who are very mindful of the needs of others; they tend to be over-full of care for children, relatives, friends, always finding something that should be put right'
Keynotes:	**Possessive or controlling hold over others**
Goal of therapy:	**Letting go, developing emotional independence**

Chicory for People: Chicory is a very powerful and important remedy for those who are possessive towards others, for those who try to bind others to them. The Chicory person needs the closeness of others for comfort and reassurance, which we all do; but they also have this need to influence and control. The Chicory person seeks affection, but is often very possessive in relationships with others, friends, family and children. They like to express their affection, but they also require a response from you. Without this response, they can withdraw and start pouting, and become offended. So there is a two-sided aspect to the Chicory state, which can alternate quite rapidly – there's the outgoing and expressive affectionate state, very giving and fussy; and there is the state of self-pity and withdrawal, looking for attention. In short, Chicory addresses the common human tendency to be self-centred, manipulative and controlling.

Chicory for Dogs: Dogs can become very expert at manipulating their owners to gain attention. Attention seeking dogs may bark, whine, stare at you, place their paw on you, climb up on top of you, and demand your undivided attention in whatever way they can! Some dogs refuse to let their owners read a book or speak on the phone, or will follow them everywhere from room to room – even to the bathroom. In some cases, when the owner tries to distance themselves from the dog to get some peace, the dog's reaction is to use whatever means at his disposal to blackmail them into doing what he wants: barking, pawing at the door, howling or even destructiveness, all designed to say 'don't you ignore me!' Eventually, worn down by the dog's tactics, the owner gives in and lets the dog have his way. The score is dog: 1 / owner: 0. The dog is learning how to get the better of you, testing the limits of your endurance and finding out the most effective ways to break your resolve.

Attention-seeking problems can be the bane of a dog-owner's life. One dog (which was later helped using Chicory) was so angry when his owner didn't pay him attention that he would bark furiously if they tried to watch TV, read a book or even look out of the window! Other ways dogs have of getting your attention include eating disorder 'protests' where the dog manipulates the owner using his refusal to eat. Owners often end up feeding the dog by hand, which just makes the attention-seeking behaviour more intense.

It's important to remember that owners have often created these tendencies in their dogs by rewarding their attention-seeking behaviour in the past; these tend to be learned behaviours that have to be unlearned through a process of teaching the dog to accept things on your terms. Chicory can help in this process, by acting to reduce the dog's urgent need to gain your attention. The remedy helps the dog to achieve greater emotional independence. There have been cases where Chicory alone was able to stop the attention-seeking behaviour altogether; in other cases the remedy's action needs to be backed up by actively paying attention to teaching the dog new habits.

Quite often, when exasperated owners are told by a dog trainer or canine behaviourist that they will have to start ignoring their dog's attention-seeking behaviours, they find that ignoring the behaviour initially just makes it worse. This is simply the dog's response to your strategy: you ignore his attempts, so he tries harder. A really determined dog can be almost impossible to ignore! Again, this is where Chicory can help, softening the dog's pressing urge to demand your attention.

Chicory is also quite important in helping separation anxiety problems, as a way of reducing the dog's stress when owners are away at work, shopping, etc. However, these can be complex and difficult problems to cure.

VERVAIN

Latin name:	Verbena officinalis
Dr Bach's words:	'They have a great wish to convert all around them to their own views of life'
Keynotes:	**Overenthusiasm, excessive exuberance, 'in your face'**
Goal of therapy:	**To restore calm, composure and sedate behaviour**

Vervain for People: According to Dr Bach's interpretation, the type of person needing Vervain often wants to convert others to their own view, to their own principles. Vervain is also a good remedy for an excessively exuberant, demonstrative and 'hyper' person.

Such people can expend huge amounts of energy when they constantly take centre stage in any social situation, talking a great deal, being very forceful with their opinions in an attempt to influence others, acting very enthusiastically towards people who agree with them. However, when they have burnt up all their energy with this hyper-exuberant behaviour, they can often withdraw into a state of exhausted tension, have angry outbursts or even become very depressed.

Vervain for Dogs: Dogs are most certainly not interested in trying to convert others to their ways! Where this remedy can help dogs is in reducing the drive of excess energy that can result in exuberance, hyperactivity and uncontrollable behaviour. When a dog acts in an apparently hyperactive way, jumps up at people, chases his tail, or never stops running about, we can try Vervain by all means but should not be too surprised if it doesn't work! There may be all sorts of factors involved: diet, training, the age and breed of the dog, and the way that people are responding to his 'hyper' behaviour. For instance, if the dog is getting rewarded by excited voices or a pat on the head each time he jumps up, this is simply teaching him that all this is a great game and a fun way of becoming the centre of attention. We can't then expect a Bach remedy to 'switch off' what we have taught him is the desired way to act. All of these factors may need to be addressed as well as using this remedy. Using Vervain in conjunction with a re-training program, e.g. gently but firmly and consistently ignoring the dog's 'hyper' behaviour is likely to bring better results than relying on the remedy alone.

The most successful Vervain cases the authors have seen in dogs have been on young pups whose overflowing energy is a more natural expression of their youthful exuberance, and less the learned behaviour typical of an older, more experienced dog.

CENTAURY

Latin Name:	Centaurium umbellatum
Dr Bach's words:	'Kind, quiet people who are over-anxious to serve others… they become more servants than willing helpers, do more than their own share of the work, and may neglect their own particular mission in life'
Keynotes:	**Weakness, the too willing servitor, the 'doormat'**
Goal of therapy:	**To restore greater assertiveness and confidence**

Centaury for People: Centaury is what could be called the 'doormat' remedy. The remedy helps people who lack confidence and have such a vulnerable state of mind that they feel they have to allow everyone to dominate them. In the Centaury state one is terribly eager to please and serve others. This is no bad thing in itself, in fact a highly commendable trait – and Centauries are often really nice, sweet people with a heart of gold. But the problem centres on the person's difficulty in asserting himself or herself and being unable to stop more forceful personalities from dominating them completely and taking them for granted. In short, Centaury is about empowerment: finding the inner strength needed to stand up for one's own freedom. Centaury doesn't take away the love of helping and serving others; instead it allows a person to find the right balance between giving to others and expecting something back in return.

Centaury for Dogs: Though there are probably some dogs that will respond to Centaury in the same kind of way they respond to other confidence-boosting remedies like Cerato and Larch, this remedy is in our experience really more of a 'people' remedy. Centaury can very much help to make dogs happier – by helping their human carers to better fit the responsible role of a good pack leader. This doesn't mean shouting or being strict with the dog all the time, it means having what it takes to bear the responsibility for the safety and strength of the pack. Someone who can't say no to people, who is too shy and retiring and never stands up for themselves, is likely to be seen by the dog as a lower-ranking pack member who could never be a leader. This often causes problems for the dog, given how heavily they depend on us for emotional security as well as food and shelter. A leaderless or weakly-led pack is a stressful environment, and the dog may feel impelled to act by taking charge. Unfortunately, the humans then turn the tables on him by refusing to tolerate certain behaviours that rightfully go hand in hand with the position of a pack leader. On the one hand they invite the dog to become their leader, then they deny him the freedom to lead them effectively. Constant mixed signals are the cause of chronic stress and confusion for millions of dogs. This only serves to highlight the importance of learning as much about canine culture and social needs as we can. If we find ourselves lacking any of the personal virtues required of a pack leader, for our dog's sake if not for our own we can help to remedy these shortcomings using a Bach flower such as Centaury.

CERATO

Latin name:	Ceratostigma willmottiana
Dr Bach's words:	'Those who have not sufficient confidence in themselves to make their own decisions. They constantly seek advice from others, and are often misguided'
Keynotes:	**Self-distrust, lack of self-belief**
Goal of therapy:	**To strengthen the personality**

Cerato for People: Cerato is a remedy for people who are hesitant with low self-confidence, who don't trust their own decisions. They will often be too reliant on other people's advice, unable to rely on their own judgement. For the same reason they often tend to be easily impressed by fads and trends, and are the kind of people to follow an opinion-leader without question. Cerato is often a good remedy for young people who have not yet developed a confident personality and may be very open to negative influences; Cerato types are often shy by nature, lacking in forcefulness and confidence. The goal of the remedy is to help boost confidence and independence. Like Centaury it helps to foster a balanced degree of assertiveness, and like Chestnut Bud it helps to mature the personality.

Cerato for Dogs: Cerato can be helpful to a young dog that lacks confidence and experience, for instance a puppy that has been taken away from his mother before she was able to teach him the important rules and 'facts of life' that a dog needs to know. This remedy can help the dog to gain more confidence in our confusing and alien human world. Other dogs that find themselves in this confusing state of mind may be dogs that have been used in intensive breeding programmes and not had very much contact with other dogs. Cerato can help them to become more sure of themselves. Another important remedy for helping dogs with a lack of confidence is Larch.

Like Centaury, Cerato can help the dog by helping his owner. People who lack confidence in themselves may have problems being seen by the dog as their leader. Because in the dog's mind every pack must have a leader, the dog with an underconfident owner will try to take on this role himself. This can lead to problems: sometimes the dog is able to do the job too well! Or else, the dog may be very stressed by the responsibility. It's important for owners to become the dog's kind, gentle but firm leader. If they feel too emotionally insecure to take on that role, Cerato is one of the Bach remedies that can help.

SCLERANTHUS

Latin name:	Scleranthus annuus
Dr Bach's words:	'Those who suffer much from being unable to decide between two things, first one seeming right then the other'
Keynotes:	**Indecisiveness, vacillation between options**
Goal of therapy:	**To restore decisive balance, clarity and focus**

Scleranthus for People: The classic use of Scleranthus in people is in helping with choices and decision-making. People needing this remedy often have trouble making up their mind between different options. There is always vacillation, or swaying, in the negative Scleranthus state. This would be the sort of person who simply can't decide whether to go to Place A or Place B for their holiday and would sit there with a brochure in each hand, staring first at one and then at the other, would decide on A and start making arrangements for that, and then would their decision and go for B, and then would change back again any number of times. Then, having travelled to Place B and sitting in their hotel room, their thoughts would start turning fretfully to what it would have been like to visit Place A instead! This chronic difficulty in deciding on a path and sticking to it can give rise to feelings of dissatisfaction, restlessness and unhappiness. Scleranthus can help the sufferer develop a more decisive and confident perspective that will improve their life generally.

Scleranthus for Dogs: This is one of those cases where the uses of the remedy are a little different than for people. Dogs generally don't suffer from indecisiveness. They're quick at making decisions once they understand the options facing them. For instance, if there's food involved and the dog works out the best and fastest way of getting it, their decision-making will be very quick indeed! Likewise, if something frightens a dog his decision to react accordingly will be instantaneous and logical: run away if possible, or stand and fight if flight isn't an option.

Thus, Scleranthus isn't so much indicated for indecisiveness in dogs, but more for other types of vacillation. There have been reported cases of Scleranthus helping dogs with physical problems that echo the Scleranthus 'swaying' tendency: these are problems such as hormonal swings, such as false pregnancies in dogs. These are imbalances where a bitch will go through all the motions of pregnancy even though not actually pregnant. She may show strange, unsettled behaviours, irritable one minute and normal the next. Scleranthus may be able to help settle these moods down.

The remedy has also been reported useful for car sickness in some dogs, nausea caused by irregular motion. This may be due to some subtle inner balancing action that the remedy is capable of, although this is still unknown in neuroscience. Note: in some cases dogs are sick in cars due to stress and nervousness, so other remedies should also be taken into account (such as Mimulus, Rock Rose and Impatiens) depending on the situation and the individual dog. When a dog is sick in the car due to a past trauma related to car travel, another important remedy is Star of Bethlehem.

Another potential use for Scleranthus is as an aid in training a dog. The remedy has the ability to help to stabilise a 'swaying' mind and so help to focus a dog's attention on the lessons you are teaching him without getting as distracted. Clear thinking, focus and decisive action are always the keywords for this remedy.

WATER VIOLET*

Latin name:	Hottonia palustris
Dr Bach's words:	'For those who in health or illness like to be alone… they are aloof, leave people alone and go their own way'
Keynotes:	**Pride, aloofness, separation from others**
Goal of therapy:	**To restore a sense of social togetherness**

Water Violet for People: Water Violet is for people who deliberately keep away from others, often because they feel superior and are reluctant to associate with them or be on the same level as them. Dr Bach noticed that Water Violet types are often very clever and talented. They may feel special or more accomplished than other people, and this talent gives them a sense of being elevated above the rest of society. But hidden behind this veneer of great self-confidence there is often a painful sense of loneliness that stems from their inability to reach out to others and feel part of a warm social togetherness. The goal of this remedy is to help melt away the barriers and allow the person to meet with others on a more equal level.

Water Violet for Dogs: The Water Violet state in dogs is less complex than in humans. With dogs, this remedy is useful in helping to re-create social harmony amongst dogs. Dogs are naturally very social animals, adapted to living in tightly organised groups that for millions of years – unlike human societies – have co-existed without problems. However, sometimes there are frictions between members of the social group if dogs are living together in a human environment. This is another reflection of the fact that dogs living in the human world are not living a very natural existence. Water Violet can help to smooth away these frictions.

The remedy can also help with what we call 'inter-species communication', creating a sense of bondedness and togetherness between dogs and people. The remedy can be used effectively with other Bach remedies like Chestnut Bud (and Clematis) for helping to train a dog, and trainers taking Water Violet together with their dogs have reported feeling as though they were 'in a bubble' together, able to communicate very closely and seeming to understand each other better, working more effectively as a team.

GENTIAN

Latin name:	Gentiana amarella
Dr Bach's words:	'Those who are easily discouraged. They may be progressing well in illness, or in the affairs of daily life, but any small delay or hindrance of progress causes doubt and soon disheartens them'
Keynotes:	**Doubt and discouragement**
Goal of therapy:	**To restore drive, determination and progress**

Gentian for People: Gentian is a remedy that works well when we lose faith or determination after a setback, or if things don't seem to improve, despite all our efforts. The negative Gentian state that comes on is a very deep sense of futility, with the belief that nothing we can do in life will ever succeed or get us anywhere. This negative attitude allows us to give up very easily in the face of even the slightest challenge. The remedy helps the person to develop greater optimism and faith, to find the strength inside them to face these challenges and develop greater stamina of the personality. The remedy is also important in states of physical illness when the person has little faith in their recovery or has doubts about the slow process of getting better. Helping to restore a positive attitude will have a beneficial effect on physical health as well, helping to promote a speedier and more complete recovery. This is another example of Dr Bach's ideas about a positive state of mind affecting the state of physical health.

Gentian helps to promote the determination we need to overcome adversity. This is nicely illustrated by an old historical story about Robert the Bruce, a Scottish warrior who fought for freedom and independence in medieval times. Hiding in a cave from English soldiers after losing a battle, Bruce felt completely defeated. Then he saw a spider making a web on the wet cave wall.

He watched how it kept falling but was never discouraged. Eventually, after many failures, it succeeded in building its web against all odd. Bruce was very inspired by this. He decided that 'if at first you don't succeed, try, try again'; which gave him the strength to overcome his pessimism and lead his armies to victory. Gentian has the same lesson to teach us.

Gentian for Dogs: Dogs, under normal circumstances, are rather similar to Bruce's spider: very resilient and not easily discouraged by challenges. However, Gentian can be very useful to a dog that has lost his vitality and drive, for instance in illness where it can help a dog that seems to be giving in to his ailment and not recovering well. It's a very good remedy to use during a dog's convalescence or at any time during his life when he needs support and strength.

Gentian is sometimes recommended for dogs and other animals that lose their appetite or suddenly become despondent. While there's no harm in considering the use of this remedy, and always check with a vet in case this change in the animal's behaviour might indicate a medical problem. If it should turn out that medical treatment is needed, Gentian is one of the Bach remedies that could be used to help the animal through the process.

ROCK ROSE*

Latin Name:	Helianthemum nummularium
Dr Bach's words:	'This is the remedy for cases when there appears no hope. In accidents or sudden illness, where the patient is very frightened or terrified, or if the condition is serious enough to cause great fear to those around.'
Keynotes:	**Acute fear/terror**
Goal of therapy:	**To restore courage and calm**

Rock Rose for People: It was discovered that the Rock Rose remedy was very effective for acute states of extreme fear and terror and their after-effects. During an acute state of terror there may be feelings of great danger, perhaps a fear of imminent death or injury, a great deal of mental turmoil and sometimes an overwhelming urge to run away. There is also a more chronic state of terror, where people feel constantly threatened, nervous and jittery. This kind of fear is distinct from the less extreme Mimulus type of anxiety, although in fact both of these fear remedies can be used together to 'cover' a fear problem from different 'angles' at once. The goal of the Rock Rose remedy is to promote courage, self control, and true heroism.

Rock Rose for Dogs: Dogs are just as capable as we are of feeling fear, both of the everyday anxiety kind (Mimulus) and of the more pressing, terrifying kind. Rock Rose can help them with great fear, terror and its after-effects. It can also help with chronic states of fearful anxiety, often seen in dogs that have been beaten or badly looked after. Dogs in this state lack confidence and show through their body language that they are very unhappy. Rock Rose is one of the remedies, together with others like Mimulus, Wild Rose, Star of Bethlehem, that can be considered in these circumstances. In acute situations, such as trying to calm down a dog that has been in an accident while waiting for the vet to arrive, Rock Rose has often been used effectively, adding a few drops to some water and moistening the dog's lips or temples. Please note: NEVER put a glass dropper in a dog's mouth, and especially not if the dog is in a state of nervous agitation or panic.

GORSE*

Latin name:	Ulex europaeus
Dr Bach's words:	'Very great hopelessness, they have given up belief that more can be done for them'
Keynotes:	**Hopelessness, apathy and despair**
Goal of therapy:	**To restore hope and the will to go on**

Gorse for People: Gorse is for very deep and powerful emotional states of hopelessness bordering on despair: a feeling of black gloom and resignation, with all hope gone. This state of mind can come on after a personal tragedy or major blow, and persist for a long time. Physically, the person may lose vitality and their incentive to live, which is a dangerous state in sickness and can lead to a rapid decline. Gorse can lift the spirits and facilitate a new, more inspiring outlook into the beyond. It's a very useful remedy also for bereavement, where grief turns to bitter nihilism and a total loss of direction.

Gorse for Dogs: These are emotional states that dogs can fall into just the same as humans. Gorse has helped many dogs suffering from deep gloom, depression and despair. They become shut off from the light, lose their will to live and survive, and can easily die if something isn't done to help them. A dog may shut down and go into this state after a loss of an owner, or if his life suddenly changes and he loses all the things that have brought comfort. Older dogs may come to need this remedy, or dogs that have suffered a traumatic experience from which they have trouble recovering psychologically.It's heartbreaking to see a dog fall into an emotional state where he doesn't care if he survives; but it's a very joyous experience to see such a dog respond to a remedy like Gorse. It's as though the light has returned, and the dog fills with the strength to go on. Gorse is a very important remedy, perhaps one of the most important.

OAK*

Latin name:	Quercus robur
Dr Bach's words:	'For those who are struggling and fighting strongly to get well… they will fight on against great difficulties, without loss of hope or effort'
Keynotes:	**Despondency from weakening resistance**
Goal of therapy:	**To restore reserves of energy and endurance**

Oak for People: Oak is a remedy able to give strength to people who despite their efforts to overcome difficulties are losing their resistance. This may be in a situation of illness, where extra strength is needed to overcome depletion and weakness; or it may apply to situations in life where circumstances, challenges or periods of hardship can affect our emotional strength.

There is a type of person who will display heroic feats of willpower, stoic determination to go on with their duties despite personal hardship and severity. As long as things go well for them, they can turn a blind eye to the pain they make themselves suffer; but as their reserves begin to dwindle – and we all have a breaking-point – setbacks and failures take their toll and feelings of futility and despondency quickly set in. Here, the Oak remedy can help them in two ways: by giving them access to fresh reserves of inner strength and also by helping them to relax their dedication to their duties and take some time to look after themselves more. This remedy works well with flower essences such as Hornbeam and Olive, which both can help to refresh our inner reserves of strength.

Oak for Dogs: Where Oak can help dogs is in building a weakened 'vital force'. Dogs, just like humans, can suffer a loss of energy and vitality as a result of a long struggle or period of deprivation. This could be a crippling illness, or a period of maltreatment or neglect. Oak can be useful in helping to rekindle vital energies and enthusiasm for life. It can be very important to use in cases where dogs are undergoing veterinary treatment, to help support their recovery. Dogs can sometimes seem to 'shut down' emotionally as a result of a severe illness or trauma, and here Oak, together with Bach remedies Gorse and Wild Rose, can really help. All these remedies can assist a dog to muster his strength in difficult times.

HEATHER

Latin name: Calluna vulgaris

Dr Bach's words: 'Those who are always seeking the companionship of anyone who may be available... they are very unhappy if they have to be left alone for any length of time'

Keynotes: **Self-preoccupation**

Goal of therapy: **To promote emotional independence**

Heather for People: Heather helps where the sufferer has problems connecting appropriately with others. You could describe the classic Heather state as 'unable to receive incoming calls'. People needing this remedy tend to be strongly self-centred and very absorbed with their own life and problems. They may feel a powerful urge to share these problems with others, in an attempt to gain attention, sympathy, or companionship. They are often very talkative, and often the listener finds themselves held there pinned, after a while probably wishing they could get away but also probably feeling guilty for wishing so! Should the listener try to bring up the issue of their own problems, the Heather type doesn't hear or doesn't connect, as they are just too preoccupied with themselves. While Heather-type behaviour may seem annoying and selfish, in many cases the only way a lonely, scared and insecure person can feel supported and understood. The saddest thing for them is that their way of forcing themselves on others can often have the opposite effect of driving those people away from them.

Heather for Dogs:　　　The essence of the Heather state in a person is mental tension with regard to their own situation and the need to express unhappiness. Dogs can need Heather too, but the way they express their need is much less neurotic and complicated.

The Heather state in a dog is a little like the Chicory state. Dogs can sometimes feel very 'left out' of our activities, and will attempt to redress the balance by gaining attention. They can be very persistent, staring or barking at you until you give in to them. This is often a learned behaviour, caused by the owner who has trained the dog to think that by acting this way they can be rewarded. Heather can't retrain the dog to think differently, but can help to reduce the mental stress and desire for attention. It's then up to the owner to teach the dog that barking or other attention-seeking behaviours are not beneficial. Many dogs suffer from separation anxiety, which is a distressing state caused by feeling unhappy at being left alone. Again, dogs should be taught to be emotionally independent and to enjoy spending time alone for reasonable periods. This can be taught to a dog. However, Heather is one remedy than can help to reduce the mental stress the dog is feeling during this time.

ROCK WATER

Latin name:	'Aqua petra'
Dr Bach's words:	'Those who are very strict in their way of living; they deny themselves many of the joys and pleasures of life because they consider it might interfere with their work'
Keynotes:	**Mental rigidity, fixed habits**
Goal of therapy:	**Learning new ways and a flexible attitude**

Rock Water for People: Rock Water is interesting because out of all Dr Bach's remedies it's the only one not prepared from a flower! Dr Bach made this remedy from a source of spring water believed to have natural healing properties.

People in need of the Rock Water remedy have a particular tendency to be very self-controlling. They need to master themselves and overcome what they see as any adverse tendencies within themselves. In theory, this could be an admirable pursuit – but the Rock Water state is out of balance, because it becomes a self-punitive one. These people become their own 'army officer'; the so-called adverse tendencies they identify within themselves include desires, longings, vital needs, normal human emotions. They suppress these things and feel themselves to be very strong and very admirable; they are proud of the effort they have made. Rock Water people, in their sense of having accomplished something really special, often want to inspire others to follow their example. They may intimidate others, sometimes alienating them but also sometimes confusing and brainwashing them, while they themselves suffer a lot of emotional strain from their self-imposed regime. The goal of the remedy is to help the person ease up on themselves, while at the same time acting with more kindness to those around.

Rock Water for Dogs: Thankfully for dogs, once again their simpler psychology allows them to avoid getting into messes such as a humans do! Where we see the Rock Water state in a dog, it's in a much less complex and neurotic form. Dogs don't feel any desire to punish themselves, deny themselves the good things in life; they don't have any interest in setting a moral example or showing everyone how wonderful they are! Nor have they any interest in trying to convert you to the way they want to live. Dogs simply are. And we humans have a lot to learn from them!

Where Rock Water can be good for dogs is in helping them with states of mental rigidity. For instance, a dog who has been used to getting his own way. The remedy can help a dog training programme to work better by helping the dog to develop a more flexible attitude towards training and new ideas. This is a way of helping to break bad habits, although it will only work if used together with positive teaching that the dog can understand. There is a saying 'you can't teach an old dog new tricks'. To some extent that's true, not just for dogs but for all of us. Our learning capacity is much more fluid when we are young, to help us learn all the many things we do at a formative stage in life. Rock Water seems to be able to help open the channels for receptivity and learning at a later stage in life, to break rigid patterns and create new pathways.

It's interesting that Rock Water, as a non-botanical subtle energy remedy, should have this effect. For those who are sceptical that plain water could be processed into a remedy like this, it's important to recognise that it isn't the water itself, but the traces of minerals from the stream, that matter. Therapists who work with crystal essences, very similar to flower remedies, find that many crystals seem to have a particular resonance with learning skills and cognitive development. And Rock Water, as a 'recording' of the subtle electrical signals of minerals and salts found in spring water, is basically a crystal essence.

VINE*

Latin name:	Vitis vinifera
Dr Bach's words:	'Very capable people, certain of their own ability, confident of success. Being so assured, they think that it would be for the benefit of others if they could be persuaded to do things as they themselves do, or as they are certain is right'
Keynotes:	**Domination of others**
Goal of therapy:	**To mellow over-assertive behaviour**

Vine for People: The mental/emotional state helped by the remedy is one of domination and control. Vine 'types' are rather like Impatiens types but are more forceful, and are often convinced of their leadership qualities and very frequently assume control over others whether or not these others are happy about it. They tend to disregard people's opinions and wishes in an overbearing way. In extreme cases, this tendency towards controlling behaviour may lead to ruthlessness or even violence as a means of staying in charge. There are also the less overtly dominant Vine types who tend to use manipulation, flattery and other tricks to help them achieve their ends. They can seem very friendly and earnest, but are no less dominating – as William Shakespeare wrote, 'a man can smile, and smile, and be a villain'. The former more dictatorial state often emerges when the latter has failed. However they express their tendencies, these people will be very goal-orientated and lacking in compassion for others. The Vine remedy helps them to regain compassion, essentially by relieving the deep fear that drives them.

Vine for Dogs: This remedy can help to mellow extremes of dominant or over-assertive behaviour in dogs. These behaviours, which can include bullying or sometimes aggressive behaviour, are inappropriate expressions of the dog's leadership role. Dogs do not become 'overdominant' like people can. The only power they want is the power of a leader who is responsible for his pack. A dog with enough confidence will try to take on that role if he sees that nobody else is doing it. Every pack needs a leader, or else it's very weak and vulnerable. In other words, his dominance isn't selfish, as human dominance so often is, but a way of trying to make the pack stronger. For this reason, Vine can't just stop a dog from being dominant – you also need to show the dog that there is no need for him to take on the leadership role. That leader should be you! Vine helps very much in this re-learning process, possibly by helping to reduce the stress the dog feels living in a leaderless pack.

The best approach to solving dominance-related behavioural problems in dogs is to take a dual approach that combines using Vine with a sensible, gentle but firm 'rank reversal' program. Many dog owners employ canine behaviourists to help them with this part of the therapy: however an excellent self-help resource is the canine behaviour videos/DVDs produced by the CFBA (Canine and Feline Behaviour Association) – see *Resources* at the end of the book.

OLIVE*

Latin name:	Olea europa
Dr Bach's words:	'Those who have suffered much mentally or physically and are so exhausted and weary that they feel they have no more strength to make any effort. Daily life is hard work for them, without pleasure'
Keynotes:	**Mental and physical weariness**
Goal of therapy:	**To restore energy and drive**

Olive for People: This remedy is for deep states of exhaustion, where people are badly in need of regeneration and extra reserves of energy. The Olive state is one where the person has reached their limits and are just too tired to go on, feeling burnt out. They may find themselves feeling unable to get excited about anything: life becomes dull and unrewarding and they may sink into sadness and apathy. The remedy helps to relieve the problem by promoting a renewal of energy and enthusiasm.

Olive for Dogs: Olive works in the same way for dogs as it does for humans. It can help to restore energy in dogs suffering from physical and mental exhaustion after a period of hardship, stress or illness, making it a useful remedy with a diverse range of potential uses. It can be helpful for rescued dogs, sick or recuperating dogs, old dogs or any dog that has been through a taxing experience and is suffering from loss of drive. Olive works very well together with Wild Rose for dogs that seem to have given up the will to go on after a very difficult experience such as a period of illness.

WILD OAT

Latin name:	Bromus ramosus
Dr Bach's words:	'Those who have ambitions to do something of prominence in their life, who wish to have much experience, and to take life to the full'
Keynotes:	**Lack of motivation and incentive**

Goal of therapy: **To catalyse, energise and move forward**

Wild Oat for People: People needing Wild Oat tend to feel unmotivated, stale and bored with their lives, feeling that they could be doing something more stimulating but often unaware how to find it or achieve it. They often don't have a calling, or they are unsure what it could be – they have trouble identifying a goal or path in their life. People needing this remedy often try several different paths but nothing seems quite right. They can become listless and frustrated, and life loses joy and sparkle for them. The remedy acts as a sort of 'rut-buster' that helps to restart their floundering system and motivates them to find a satisfying new direction, or else give a boost to an old one gone stale.

Wild Oat for Dogs: Wild Oat is so well known as the 'career/ life path remedy' that it's easy to get sidetracked by this view when it comes to considering its role in canine care. it would be absurd to suggest that Wild Oat could help a dog figure out what he wanted to do with his life! Dogs don't have problems about their career path or what motivates them in life. As long as they have the basic needs of company, shelter and most importantly food, they are generally happy. Dogs just want to be dogs, and they need no remedies to help them achieve 'dogness'.

What they do occasionally need, though, is a helping hand at times when they lack drive and energy in their lives. Essentially, Wild Oat's action is as a catalyst and energiser, helping to create new pathways for moving forward – and this is how to regard this remedy for the purposes of canine care. Dr Bach observed that giving this remedy could enhance the actions of other Bach flowers. He noticed that where a case was 'stuck' or there was lack of progress in treatment, adding Wild Oat to the chosen list of remedies could act to unblock the process. If, for instance, a dog was generally down and lacking in drive and energy, adding Wild Oat to a blend of remedies such as Oak, Olive, Hornbeam, Wild Rose and Gentian may help to create a more dynamic effect. Remember, though, always to have your dog checked by the vet if he shows a sudden drop in energy levels, vitality and joy of living. Should this turn out to have some medical cause, the Bach remedies can still be used alongside any other treatment.

Another important use of Wild Oat in canine care is in helping dogs indirectly by making their owners happier and more satisfied with life. Having to live with someone who suffers from a negative Wild Oat state could be very stressful for a dog. If the person helped themselves with this or any other needed remedy, the benefits they felt would also act to reduce the 'sponge effect' or secondary stress felt by the dog.

CHERRY PLUM*

Latin name:	Prunus cerasifera
Dr Bach's words:	'Fear of the mind being over-strained, of reason giving way, of doing fearful and dreaded things... there comes the thought and impulse to do them'
Keynotes:	**Fear of losing mental balance**
Goal of therapy:	**To restore calm, balance and inner peace**

Cherry Plum for People: In the Cherry Plum state, the mind is overstrained and out of balance, with a sense of struggling against itself. A Cherry Plum state can come on during a period of stress, when we feel like cracking and may fall in a heap of tears, or else have a fit of rage and smash something that we will regret later! Cherry Plum can be of use in nervousness, shyness, and stage fright, these being unwanted mental states where one tries to fight against oneself. Cherry Plum has also often helped more serious emotional states where sufferers feel severe internal pressure that influences their behaviour. It's an effective remedy where there is frightening loss of control – it's useful in drug or alcohol rehabilitation, obsessive-compulsive disorders, and many types of behaviour that might be reckless, impulsive and risky. Some psychologists have used the remedy to help patients with self-destructive tendencies. Cherry Plum's goal is to reduce pressure from the unconscious, to give mental peace and relaxation.

Cherry Plum for Dogs: Once again we see that, luckily for dogs, they don't fall prey to the same depths of mental torment as humans. However, dogs are capable, at a certain level, of experiencing mental/emotional stress that can push them over the edge. Cherry Plum helps dogs suffering from extremes of stress that create erratic thought processes, hysterical or aggressive behaviour. The remedy can help to bring calm in frightening situations that threaten to tip the dog's mind into panic or loss of control.

Note: In cases of aggression in dogs, never rely entirely on this or any other form of natural therapy. The dog should always be seen by a veterinary surgeon and/or a qualified canine behaviourist. The authors recommend that canine behaviourists or behaviour counsellors who advise dog owners to give psychotropic drugs (e.g. Prozac and Valium) to their animals should be avoided.

ELM*

Latin name:	Ulmus procera
Dr Bach's words:	'At times there may be periods of depression when they feel that the task they have undertaken is too difficult, and not within the power of a human being'
Keynotes:	**Overwhelm, loss of will**
Goal of therapy:	**Ability to deal calmly with pressure**

Elm for People: Elm is for states of being overwhelmed and subdued by tasks, duties or responsibilities that seem to loom over us and appear insolvable. The more we focus on the problem, the less we are able to focus on the solution: this becomes a vicious circle that may start a decline into great mental stress, even despair and despondency. It may be a sign that the sufferer has been working too hard and needs to rest; after a break the mind may perceive things differently. The goal of the Elm remedy is to help the mind to relax and step back from things and gain a fresher perspective. The remedy helps to organise the mind, to give it clarity and to allow a person to grow beyond their troubles.

Elm for Dogs: Dogs can become very overwhelmed and mentally stressed by too many impressions happening at once. They are perfectly adapted to the slower, more focused pace of nature, but our modern human society can be very bewildering to them. Dogs that have to live in chaotic or stressful environments such as hectic cities, kennels or rescue centres, can become confused and unhappy due to the sensory overload. Though of course we need to do everything possible to reduce the amount of stress a dog has to deal with, Elm can additionally help the dog by relaxing his mind in the face of all these potentially troubling impressions.

Similarly, Elm can also be very helpful in puppy socialisation, where young dogs are introduced for the first time to the many things they have to learn to deal with in life. Giving Elm to the dog for a period of time can be a major help through this process, helping to prevent the youngster from becoming overwhelmed by all the new sense impressions such as busy streets, rooms full of unknown people, and crowded puppy classes. It's important that a dog should make positive associations with all these things early in life, as a dog that is allowed to become frightened by early socialisation experiences will often grow up to become a fearful adult. Poor socialisation is one of the key reasons for dogs to attack strangers in later life and end up having to be destroyed under public safety legislation. Another important remedy to aid socialisation is Walnut, along with courage and confidence-giving remedies such as Larch, Mimulus and Cerato.

Elm can also be useful in training a dog, to help him to learn and assimilate information without becoming confused. Another useful remedy to help in a similar way is Chestnut Bud.

ASPEN*

Latin name:	Populus tremula
Dr Bach's words:	'Vague unknown fears, for which there can be given no explanation, no reason... yet the patient may be terrified of something terrible going to happen'
Keynotes:	**Fears of unclear or unconscious origin**
Goal of therapy:	**Confidence and courage**

Aspen for People: Aspen deals with a particular kind of fear that needs to be distinguished from Mimulus or Rock Rose-type fears. People in need of Aspen are fearful, often with a sense of hovering anxiety, an undercurrent of panic, but they have difficulty understanding the root of their fear. An Aspen-type fear is more mysterious than a simple fear of a thing, place, person, or experience. It's often linked to supernatural or metaphysical fears from the unconscious, or a deep psychological fear of the unknown that may be reflected in the person's dreams. Deep fears of the unknown, of the future, of what lies beyond death, are all glimpses of the workings of our unconscious mind. If we are unconsciously full of tension and anxiety, this will tend to filter through to the conscious mind as this nebulous, undefined Aspen-type nervousness. The remedy, then, addresses fears that we may not even be fully aware of consciously, helping to make life easier by relieving that inner burden.

Aspen for Dogs: Dogs normally will always have a clear idea what they are afraid of. For instance if there is a certain person they fear, when that person comes into the room the dog may start to act fearfully or give that person 'calming signals' to say 'I am not a threat to you'. Animals do not, as far as we know, have the same kind of unconscious or metaphysical fears that we more complex humans have. These facts tend to indicate that we are less likely to see the classic Aspen-type fears affecting dogs.

However, this doesn't mean that Aspen cannot be a useful remedy for dogs. Some types of fear in dogs can be helped with Aspen – for instance when a dog is old, or ill, and the unconscious sense of his declining physical state makes him feel vulnerable. In this situation a dog can lose confidence and start to appear nervous although there's nothing directly frightening him. Aspen isn't a treatment for whatever illness may be affecting the dog, but can support his state of mind and help give strength to aid in recovery. Old dogs can be helped to feel happier and more confident in their last phase of life.

CHESTNUT BUD*

Latin name:	Aesculus hippocastanum
Dr Bach's words:	'For those who do not take full advantage of observation and experience, and who take a longer time than others to learn the lessons of daily life... they find themselves having to make the same error on different occasions when once would have been enough'
Keynotes:	**Immaturity, inability to learn from mistakes**
Goal of therapy:	**Increased focus and learning ability**

Chestnut Bud for People: Chestnut Bud is a remedy for those who find themselves making the same mistakes again and again, as though they never learned from their errors. In this state the mind is restless and impulsive, not fully engaged in the here and now. A person in need of this remedy tends to be easily distracted, absent minded, and often with a certain tendency to immaturity. Chestnut Bud is very often used for learning disabilities and problems faced by young people who find it hard to concentrate, often because of difficulty focusing on the present. This results in their being unable to retain information from lessons and life experience, so that they often appear to stumble from one situation to another without seeming to learn from life. People who need Chestnut bud are often driven by their emotions, failing to reason carefully and reflect on the effect of their actions and words. The remedy, taken over time, can help to reverse this tendency by allowing for better retention of lessons, whether taught in the classroom or in the 'school of life'.

Chestnut Bud for Dogs: Chestnut Bud works for the dogs in much the same way it does for people. This remedy is often useful in helping young animals that act quite impulsively and may be prone to making the same mistakes over and over. The remedy helps to increase focus and reduce the excessive spontaneity of their actions, encouraging more rational thought and concentration. Dogs are capable of clear rational thinking, especially when this ability is well encouraged and stimulated. Animals in need of this remedy tend to be easily distracted, lacking in attention span and often forgetting the lessons of their training. Chestnut Bud has been observed to help these animals to listen more carefully and retain their lessons better. Many dog trainers, including a number of professionals, have found that using Chestnut Bud helps them get better results, especially with those dogs that might normally present more of a challenge due to their scatty, impulsive natures.

Chestnut Bud is also a very useful remedy alongside Walnut, Elm, Larch, Cerato and Mimulus in helping young dogs and puppies with their early learning and socialisation.

LARCH*

Latin name:	Larix decidua
Dr Bach's words:	'For those who do not consider themselves as good or capable as those around them, who expect failure, who feel that they will never be a success, and so do not venture or make a strong enough attempt to succeed'
Keynotes:	**Low self-confidence**
Goal of therapy:	**Emotional security and self-assurance**

Larch for People:　　Larch is for states of low self-confidence, a problem that affects most people at some time, and can cause a great deal of suffering. Poor confidence can stifle a person's whole life, sapping energy, spoiling relationships, stunting personal growth and putting them off trying anything new as they are convinced in advance that they would fail. People needing Larch have the tendency to compare themselves to others, always unfavourably so that they always see themselves as in some way inferior. A chronic lack of confidence may feel like a mild depression, where life holds no joy and the sufferer has no drive to do anything about it. In such instances Larch can be combined with other remedies such as Wild Rose, Wild Oat, and Mustard.

Larch for Dogs:　　There are many circumstances where a dog can suffer from a lowered sense of self-confidence. Dogs can lose confidence in old age, when they feel their strength, social status and ability to survive in the wild begin to slip away. At the other end of the age scale, a young dog can feel underconfident and insecure, especially if he hasn't been thoroughly socialised. A dog that is ill may fall into a nervous, anxious and insecure state of mind. Dogs that are stressed by their environment, for instance by living with unhappy people, can also suffer a loss of confidence. So Larch can work in many situations, and together with many other Bach remedies depending on the circumstances.

HORNBEAM*

Latin name:	Carpinus betulus
Dr Bach's words:	'For those who feel that they have not sufficient strength, mentally or physically, to carry the burden of life placed upon them... who believe that some part, of mind or body, needs to be strengthened'
Keynotes:	**Mental fatigue and loss of concentration**
Goal of therapy:	**Restored mental energy and focus**

Hornbeam for People: This is a strengthening remedy for those times when the mind feels washed out, overtired and unable to concentrate any longer. The Hornbeam state often results from a period of hard work, especially mental work such as intense research or academic studies. Many students find themselves needing this remedy, to help with revision before an exam when their brains are crammed with information. Anyone who faces a challenge, perhaps running a business, may sometimes need to refresh their tired mind using Hornbeam. People needing the remedy often feel unable to rise to their tasks any longer, badly in need of a mental and physical energy boost. The mind can become hazy and unfocused, listless and inefficient. The remedy helps to access reserves of mental energy, allowing greater focus and concentration.

Hornbeam for Dogs: Hornbeam can be an important remedy to help dogs through periods of stress or illness. In just the same way that it can help people, it can help dogs to become more alive, alert and focused. It's one of the Bach remedies that can help maintain vital energy when a dog needs it most, for instance during convalescence or in fighting a serious illness. As Dr Bach wisely observed, the patients with the low mental energy or downcast spirits are the ones who often tend to cope less well.

If your dog suddenly starts acting very lethargically and seems mildly depressed, always check with the vet that there's nothing medically wrong. Hornbeam has been known to help many dogs in a weak or vulnerable state, but it isn't a cure for the illness itself.

WILLOW

Latin name:	Salix vitellina
Dr Bach's words:	'For those who have suffered adversity or misfortune and find these difficult to accept without resentment... they feel that they have not deserved so great a trial, that it was unjust, and they become embittered'
Keynotes:	**Resentment and bitterness**
Goal of therapy:	**Ability to let go of negative feelings**

Willow for People: This remedy treats states of resentment, against other people, circumstances or life in general. This state can linger for years, and its sufferers can fall into a very depressed and despondent state. They can also become bitter and blame others for their unlucky lot in life. Often, the failure may lie with the person themselves and their feelings are quite unfounded. In other cases there may be a real reason for their sense of bitterness. Either way it's a very damaging negative emotional burden. The remedy helps the person to let go of this feeling, allowing them to put the past behind them and start afresh with a clearer mind.

Willow for Dogs: In dogs, Willow helps with a sense of resentment against specific others, or against humans in general, perhaps as a result of maltreatment. Sometimes a dog seems to dislike or resent people or a specific person, and it may be that certain people may be frightening the dog without realising it; also the dog may be reminded of someone who was unkind in the past. This is often the case with rescued dogs. There are other Bach remedies we need to learn about to help with these kinds of cases, most notably Star of Bethlehem, an extremely important remedy we talk about later in the book.

Dogs can also harbour grudges as a result of hierarchy displacement. That is to say, they can become jealous when attention that was theirs is suddenly switched to someone else. Examples of this include a new puppy coming into the household, or a new baby. Willow is one remedy that has been known to help dogs with their feelings of resentment against the newcomer. Another remedy is Holly to help with jealousy. You should back this up by taking some time to pay special attention to the dog for at least a few minutes each day.

Important note: do NOT rely on Willow or any other type of remedy to deal with any situation where a jealous dog could potentially pose a risk to, for instance, a baby or young child. Always seek the help of a professional canine behaviourist. The authors recommend the CFBA (Canine/Feline Behaviour Association) for any such problems.

BEECH*

Latin name:	Fagus sylvatica
Dr Bach's words:	'To have the ability to see the good within… to be more tolerant, more lenient, and understanding'
Keynotes:	**Intolerance and annoyance**
Goal of therapy:	**Opening up to tolerance and compassion**

Beech for People: The Beech remedy helps those who are overly critical and intolerant of others, always seeking to guide and shape other people's will. They have a very negative outlook, and to be in their presence is a very taxing, tiring, demanding experience. We all know people like this, who demand such high standards from everyone or seem to believe they're always right. It's a state of arrogance, constantly finding fault and highly judgmental.

The Beech state, though it's exasperating and annoying in another person, is actually a sad one, and there's often some underlying reason for its development. In many cases such a state comes on after a trauma such as shock, letdown or grief, if this hasn't been properly dealt with. The Beech attitude is also sometimes a means of self-defensive 'armouring', where the person mounts a shield between themselves and others. Beech lessens the tendency to criticise, and opens the mind up to tolerance and acceptance, to get in touch with hidden sadness and experiences that have not been released or dealt with.

Beech for Dogs: Because the dog's mind is much less complex than ours, we only see the Beech state in a very simplified form. Dogs aren't arrogant or judgmental, negative or intolerant. However, one important use for Beech in dogs is to help those animals that have become untrusting of people as a result of unpleasant experiences. When all a dog has ever known of humans is fear, maltreatment, pain, loneliness and discomfort, he learns not to like or trust us. His unfriendly behaviour is simply a way of protecting himself from a type of animal (us) that experience has taught him is hostile and to be avoided. These kinds of traits are often seen in dogs that have been abandoned or have run wild and end up in the dog 'rescue' system. Rescue organisations try to find the dogs homes with caring families, but their behaviour can make it hard for them to adjust to life with people. Beech is one remedy that can helps to soften their hardened attitude and help them learn to trust again.

Note: it isn't wise to trust Beech, or any flower remedy, in the case of a dog that has turned aggressive. Be very careful if you are taking in a rescue dog, in case of potentially dangerous aggression problems. Remember that even a small dog can badly injure an adult and easily kill a child.

CRAB APPLE*

Latin Name:	Malus pumila/Malus sylvestris
Dr Bach's words:	'This is the remedy of cleansing. For those who feel as if they had something not quite clean about themselves'
Keynotes:	**Personal shame or disgust**
Goal of therapy:	**Cleansing, acceptance, self-esteem**

Crab Apple for People: This remedy helps people who suffer from shameful feelings about themselves. They often feel a deep sense of uncleanness, either relating to the way they look, the way they feel, or things that they have done – 'dirty', shameful actions. We are not talking strictly about guilt here – the emphasis tends to be on personal, often physical, shame, a strong dislike of some aspect of the person that they feel is nasty, unwholesome or ugly.

Crab Apple is also useful for humans feeling shocked or disgusted after dealing with nasty things. For instance, whether you are a veterinary nurse or a dog owner, looking after a very sick dog can be a hard experience, even if it's a dog you really love. You may be exposed to tasks, sights and smells that are not nice. Crab Apple can help to 'cleanse' these unpleasant impressions from your mind.

Crab Apple for Dogs: Dogs don't, as far as anyone knows, suffer from 'poor body image' or the feelings of shame, self-hatred and disgust that some unhappy humans do. Dogs are lucky enough to be free of such painful neuroses. However, that doesn't mean we should disregard this remedy for canine use. Crab Apple has some useful physical applications for dogs. Research has shown that combined with the other Bach remedies Cherry Plum and Impatiens, it can have a very good effect on skin problems. This effective combination is contained within the 'Rescue' Cream that is easily available from stores. This is the easiest and best way to use Crab Apple for such problems. It can help with allergic reactions such as 'hot spots' in dogs, minor wounds and grazes that do not require the vet's attention, burns and stings. In itchy skin conditions where the dog is always scratching and damaging the skin, the cream can help to reduce the urge to scratch while promoting healing.

WALNUT*

Latin name:	Juglans regia
Dr Bach's words:	'The remedy gives constancy and protection from outside influences'
Keynotes:	**Impressionability from outside influences**
Goal of therapy:	**Protection and stability**

Walnut for People: Walnut is an important and frequently-used remedy that helps with oversensitivity to outside impressions. This oversensitivity can manifest itself in a variety of ways: the Walnut 'type' may be over-susceptible to stress or upset in chaotic situations, and some people are easily prone to suffer after observing sad events or shocking news items on TV or unpleasant scenes in films. Walnut can help to reduce the intensity of their reactions to these influences.

Another manifestation of a negative Walnut state is where the person tends to be too easily swayed or influenced. This is similar to the Cerato state: they may be too easily taken by trends and fads, or too easily attracted to certain persons or movements. The remedy helps to promote the independence needed to detach oneself from these influences and gain a healthy distance from them.

Walnut for Dogs: Walnut is an important remedy for dogs. It can help in two basic ways. The first way Walnut helps is by offering strength during times of change. Dogs are creatures that thrive on a consistent and healthy routine. They don't like change, unless of course it's a nice new blanket to lie on or an especially tasty new kind of food! The changes that threaten dogs are changes of territory or changes in the social group. When families move home, dogs can be quite unsettled. Walnut can help them to readjust to the new home. You should also do everything you can to make the dog feel comfortable, by giving him a place with his familiar old bed for instance. When a new pack member arrives, such as a new dog, new baby, new husband or wife, Walnut is one of the remedies that can help the dog to readjust to the change. The same applies to when a pack member leaves or dies (the same, in the dog's mind). In different cases, different remedies will also be needed to help depending on the situation.

The other basic way Walnut can be useful for a dog is by helping him to assimilate his environment. It can be helpful in socialising a young puppy, assisting him to take on board all the new experiences around him. Walnut is also important in situations where a dog's living environment is stressful, for instance living with a quarrelsome or unhappy family. This is extremely difficult for the dog. We mentioned earlier in the book that Agrimony can help here; Walnut is another useful Bach remedy in these cases. It's also highly important to reduce the levels of stress, argument or unhappiness in the household.

HOLLY*

Latin name:	Ilex aquifolium
Dr Bach's words:	'For those who sometimes are attacked by thoughts of such kind as jealousy, envy, revenge and suspicion... for the different forms of vexation'
Keynotes:	**Vexation, annoyance and jealousy**
Goal of therapy:	**Compassion, tolerance and serenity**

Holly for People: Holly is another important and frequently-needed Bach remedy. Again, this remedy is concerned with how we cope with stress, and how life's experiences have shaped and moulded our personality. The person in need of Holly tends to overreact to any disturbance by becoming irascible and angry. Sometimes these overreactions are extremely powerful and violent, with outbursts of rage, physical aggressiveness, abuse, and impulsive or erratic behaviour. Less overt but just as psychologically destructive manifestations of this mental state are simmering hatred, jealousy and possessiveness.

Holly for Dogs: Holly can also help dogs with feelings of jealousy and vexation. These can be triggered by a variety of things. One example is when a new puppy is brought into the household and older dogs feel resentful towards him. This situation should always be carefully handled, but Holly can help the process of acceptance. Jealousy problems sometimes emerge when a couple have a new baby and suddenly stop paying attention to their dog. Depending on the dog's individual personality, he may respond by becoming withdrawn and depressed, or he may start to look for ways to gain attention, or else he may become jealous and hostile. In one case, a dog stole a baby from a cot when the mother wasn't looking, took it outside and attempted to bury it in the garden! Luckily the infant was completely unharmed. The dog shouldn't really be blamed for this behaviour, as jealousy is only his normal reaction to the circumstances: in canine logic, removing the baby is just a way of making things go back to the way they were before. Bach remedies Holly (or Willow, for resentment) can help to reduce the intensity of the dog's reaction. However, it's important in these situations to take some time out and play with the dog for at least a few minutes each day to prevent him from feeling left out.

You will sometimes read in Bach flower books that Holly will reduce aggression in dogs. While it's true that Holly can sometimes have a 'mellowing' effect on some cases, in general this is something of an over-simplification of canine aggression. And because of the serious nature of this problem, such an over-simplification could be dangerous.

Remember that dogs are pragmatists: they never do anything without a reason. If they act aggressively this is because they are afraid, or because they are trying to protect some resource such as food or territory. Another resource they will protect is their place in the pack, and anything that threatens that may be a target for aggressive behaviour if the dog feels confident enough. Their behaviour isn't an emotional imbalance or an irrational action, and so it would be wrong to say that a remedy can just stop the behaviour. The best 'remedy' is to understand why the dog is acting aggressively and to take steps to make sure that he no longer needs to behave this way. This can be a very difficult and complex type of behaviour problem to fix, and it can also be dangerous as an aggressive dog can do a lot of damage. For these reasons, ordinary dog owners are not advised to try to deal with aggression problems on their own, and should not rely on a remedy like Holly (or Cherry Plum, Willow, etc.) to stop the behaviour. You need to work with a good canine behaviourist in these cases. The authors recommend the CFBA (Canine and Feline Behaviour Association), who are actively opposed to the use of any form of behaviour-altering drugs in canine behaviour therapy.

STAR OF BETHLEHEM*

Latin name:	Ornithogalum umbellatum
Dr Bach's words:	'For those in great distress, great unhappiness, the shock of serious news, the loss of someone dear, the fright following an accident… those who for a time refuse to be consoled'
Keynotes:	**Sadness, shock, grief, past trauma**
Goal of therapy:	**Overcoming past hurts, moving on**

Star of Bethlehem for People: This is an extremely important Bach remedy that helps with sadness and despair, emotional trauma and shock. Star of Bethlehem is very effective in black, grim situations of loss and bereavement, the sudden death of a loved one or some other devastating impact that seems to tear our world apart.

Star of Bethlehem is also very effective as a retro-active therapy to help with trauma that lies back in the past, even as far back as childhood. As the release happens there may be dreams or emerging memories of the traumatic event. This is one of the more amazing properties of Star of Bethlehem, its ability to help people process emotional pain that has been buried for years and may even have been forgotten. In one case, a man in his 30s who had a phobia of water was cured with Star of Bethlehem. In dreams he remembered that as a small child he had nearly drowned. He couldn't remember this happening, so asked his mother. She confirmed that he had had a very serious near-death accident in water at the age of 3, which she had never wanted to remind him about as he seemed to have pushed it from his conscious mind. The Bach flower therapy was able to help with the upper 'layer' of the problem, his fears, but at a deeper level it removed from his unconscious mind the psychological scar that was causing the pain. There have been many, many such cases with this remarkable remedy. In another case, a woman who had suffered from depression ever since coming home to find her husband dead in the bath was cured after Star of Bethlehem was added to her therapy. She began to dream about the incident and was able to weep for the first time. As the daughter of a very strict soldier she had been brought up not to show emotions, and it was the buried emotional pain that was causing the depression. As she was able to release the pain, so the depression lifted. After 7 years it had not returned. Star of Bethlehem is perhaps one of the most important remedies in Dr Bach's entire repertoire.

Star of Bethlehem for Dogs: Star of Bethlehem works in very much the same way for dogs as it does for people, and is one of the most important remedies in the entire Bach collection when it comes to canine care. One of its key uses is in canine rescue, to help with the rehabilitation and emotional healing of traumatised, psychologically-scarred dogs. The authors have often recommended that Star of Bethlehem should be given to any dog with an uncertain past, to help with any past problems that may have left a mark on the dog's present state of mind. Unfortunately, many dogs suffer very bad treatment at the hands of humans, so 'past trauma' frequently involves maltreatment from past owners. Traumatic incidents can befall even the best cared-for dog: accidents in the car, attacks from other dogs, and so on. Whatever the cause, these are events that have a deep effect on the dog. Research has found that even if you give the remedies to treat the obvious emotional problem, such as a remedy for fear (e.g. Rock Rose or Mimulus), you often will not get full results until you also address the underlying traumatic incident. This is where Star of Bethlehem is extremely beneficial. Due to its uncanny ability to 'reach back in time' and address traumas that may have happened years before, it can help many dogs whose problems all started after the unpleasant incident or period of their life happened to them.

WHITE CHESTNUT

Latin name:	Aesculus hippocastanum
Dr Bach's words:	'For those who cannot prevent thoughts, ideas, arguments which they do not desire from entering their minds... thoughts which worry and will remain and cause mental torture'
Keynotes:	**Lack of mental tranquillity**
Goal of therapy:	**Restoration of inner peace**

White Chestnut for People: White Chestnut helps with a problem most of us have experienced in adulthood, if not as children. This is the feeling of having seemingly endless trains of unwanted thought spinning round and round inside one's head: maybe thoughts about bills or things that need mending, or things that are wrong with family relationships, problems at work, problems with the car... the list is endless. Life is complex and full of niggling worries for most people, but for someone who needs White Chestnut it's even worse, as they are unable to switch these thoughts off and relax. A very tense state can develop, resulting in insomnia and a damaging impact on daily life. Left untreated over time, this worried state of mind can end up causing physical problems such as stomach ulcers, irritable colon or skin disorders. The goal of the remedy is to help open up the mind to release that strenuous pressure. White Chestnut helps to dissolve this nagging feeling of worry, and restores inner peace to set the mind free.

White Chestnut for Dogs: The promotion of mental tranquillity is just as important for dogs as it is for humans. Dogs can suffer enormously from stressful states of mind, even if they don't (as far as we know) consciously work thoughts and ideas over in their mind. The remedy addresses the same underlying mental tension that affects our two species slightly differently. A dog that seems agitated, restless, unable to settle, constantly fidgeting or shifting about, may often benefit from this remedy's calming virtues. It's also important to check that no physical problem or discomfort is making the dog feel restless.

RED CHESTNUT

Latin name:	Aesculus carnea
Dr Bach's words:	'For those who find it difficult not to be anxious for other people... they may suffer much, frequently anticipating that some unfortunate thing may happen to them'
Keynotes:	**Fear for others' welfare**
Goal of therapy:	**Emotional independence**

Red Chestnut for People: This remedy addresses a fear for the welfare of others. A person needing Red Chestnut has a tendency to worry excessively about their loved ones, often finding themselves imagining the worst things that could befall them. Often the nature of the state is that they are out of reach of that person, unable to help, powerless. This is the classic Red Chestnut fear: the other person is in need, and there is this rising fear that something horrible will happen to them. This very unnerving feeling of apprehension is often experienced by parents with small children, though it can also apply to many other situations. The goal of the remedy isn't to stop being a concerned parent, but rather to develop the ability to step back and have faith that everything will be all right. The message of this remedy is that life is too short to spend it worrying for no good reason!

Red Chestnut for Dogs: Red Chestnut is also needed in canine care, though in a slightly different way. The negative Red Chestnut state can arise in dogs that have become too closely bonded to someone. This person is often their owner, who has allowed the dog to become too emotionally dependent on them. When the owner has to go away, for instance while they are at work during the day, the dog may become very stressed and anxious. Red Chestnut has a role to play in helping to reduce this anxiety. It's also important to teach the dog to become more emotionally independent, in order to prevent separation problems from occurring in the first place. This is quite easily done by not allowing the dog to follow you around everywhere. For more information on separation anxiety problems, see the section on this subject later in the book.

Red Chestnut is an example of how the uses of Bach remedies for humans can mislead us to think too anthropomorphically if we aren't careful. For instance, one published book on Bach remedies for animals takes the remedy too literally by suggesting that it can make a mother cat less protective of her kittens. This is a misunderstanding of animal behaviour and how the remedies work. Any animal mother will naturally protect her young from a threat, such as a predator or someone who may want to harm the babies. Mother dogs with young puppies naturally want to protect them, and will if necessary defend them with aggression. No amount of Red Chestnut will stop this natural behaviour!

Note: while we are on this subject, the reader should always be aware that if they find themselves together with a bitch and her young puppies, they should always be very careful not to get too close to the pups. To allow the bitch to think you are a threat could be a safety hazard.

PINE

Latin name:	Pinus sylvestris
Dr Bach's words:	'For those who blame themselves. Even when successful they think that they could have done better... they suffer much from the faults they attach to themselves'
Keynotes:	**Guilt and self-blame**
Goal of therapy:	**Acceptance and freedom from regret**

Pine for People: Pine is the Bach remedy that deals with one of the most painful and destructive emotions we know: guilt and regret. Guilt, or a sense of having failed or done wrong, places a terrible burden on the heart and heavy strain on our whole being. It can become impossible to find inner peace, and many sufferers become depressed and despondent.

People needing Pine may be feeling guilty for a real reason – there may be real deeds of wrongdoing they are responsible for, and they are troubled by the memory. In other cases blame may be taken on board by someone who is actually quite innocent, for instance if you blame yourself that an accident was your fault. In one Pine case, the wife of a stroke victim blamed herself that she didn't do enough to push her husband to seeing the doctor, or stop smoking and drinking so much. Another man was tormented because years before during a childhood game, his brother had been killed falling out of a tree onto railings. It was not his fault, but he had always blamed himself for his brother's death. Whether you were responsible or not, guilt can be a very destructive emotion. Pine helps to let go of the past, while making amends. It allows a person to experience self-forgiveness, or to assess objectively whether or not they really can blame themselves for something. The ultimate goal, as always, is a lightness of the inner self and a good balance of the emotions.

Pine for Dogs: The most important factor in examining Pine for dogs is that, as far as we can tell, they don't feel guilt. This is one state of mind that they don't appear to share with us. Some owners insist that their dogs have 'a guilty look' when they do something naughty, like raid the garbage bin. The dog will look up at you, frowning, and he can look like the guilty expression on a person's face. But a dog that looks unhappy when you catch him doing something naughty, such as stealing food or raiding the garbage, doesn't look that way because he feels guilty. Instead, what the dog is probably thinking is that you are about to punish him, yell or shout and send him to bed – or, if the dog has been mistreated by people in the past, he may think you're going to kick or beat him. So this isn't a guilty state, but an anxious, fearful one. The dog is worried, stressed; and if you watch closely you will see he's probably giving you calming signals such as licking his lips and nose and assuming a submissive body posture. These canine calming signals are part of a dog's language. The signals say 'I'm no threat to you, please don't hurt me'. This is the dog's attempt to try to 'switch off' your aggressive behaviour towards him. The sad thing is that most people can't read the calming signals and continue to shout at the dog, which is stressful and confusing.

So Pine is really more a 'people' remedy. Dog owners sometimes need it in those sad circumstances when dogs are very old or sick, or badly injured, and have to be put to sleep by the vet. People go through a range of sad emotions when a pet dies, and one of the emotions can be guilt. People may feel they didn't do the right thing, or sometimes they start thinking about what they should have done to look after the dog better while he was alive. Most of these feelings are irrational, especially if you have been a caring and kind owner. But guilt hurts whether it's justified or not, and Pine can be an important remedy in these difficult times. By taking the remedy, people can come to an understanding that there was nothing they did wrong and nothing they could have done better, or, if they did do something wrong and, say, a preventable accident was the cause of the dog's death, they can be helped to find self-forgiveness whilst making sure the mistake doesn't happen again.

HONEYSUCKLE*

Latin name:	Lonicera caprifolium
Dr Bach's words:	'Those who live in the past, perhaps a time of great happiness, or memories of a lost friend, or ambitions which have not come true. They do not expect further happiness such as they have had'
Keynotes:	**Longing for past happiness, nostalgia**
Goal of therapy:	**Letting go of the past, looking forward**

Honeysuckle for People: The Honeysuckle remedy helps people whose minds tend to dwell too much in the past. They are detached from the present, and also from the future, often believing that the best times of their lives are behind them and the present and future hold no possibility for happiness. Such people may want to show you old photographs or tell nostalgic stories from the past, always dwelling on events from long ago. There's often a kind of dreaminess to the Honeysuckle state, but where the dreamy Clematis state gazes out to the future thinking 'one day I'll be happy', Honeysuckle looks back thinking 'I was happy then'. The Honeysuckle remedy helps to ease this sad state of mind by helping to promote a sense of optimism for the present and the future.

One of Honeysuckle's major uses is in helping to heal the heartbreak after losing a loved one, where it works very well with other remedies such as Star of Bethlehem and Gorse. It's also a key remedy for helping the problems of the elderly, who often slip into a backward-looking state of mind where they are making no effort to enjoy life any longer. The goal of the remedy is to allow a person to continue holding on to past joys and happy memories, while at the same time opening up to the potential for life in the present and the future to bring more happiness.

Honeysuckle for Dogs: Honeysuckle is quite an important remedy for dogs. Just as it can help humans after a painful loss of a loved one, it can help dogs that have lost their joy of life after losing a friend, companion or owner. We have already learned that Gorse can help dogs that have lost their spark of happiness after such a sad event. Honeysuckle is another remedy that can be used to help dogs recover emotionally and move on.

Honeysuckle is also an important remedy to help with problems of separation anxiety, a common problem that we'll be returning to later. It occurs when dogs are left on their own for a period of time, feeling stressed as a result. To the dog, this creates the same emotional pain as though their owner had died, even if it's only for a short time. Honeysuckle can help the dog to become more emotionally independent. There are also training and behaviour programmes to help this process.

WILD ROSE*

Latin name: Rosa canina

Dr Bach's words: 'Those who become resigned to all that happens without any effort to improve things and find some joy... they have surrendered to the struggle of life without complaint'

Keynotes: **Apathy, resignation, giving up the struggle**

Goal of therapy: **Courage and determination to survive**

Wild Rose for People: Wild Rose is another important remedy, helping in situations of such unhappiness and emotional hardship that the sufferer feels paralysed, unable to rise above their problems any longer. It's a state of apathy, despondency and resignation to one's fate, all energy spent, resistance seeming futile. The person may start to withdraw into themselves, as though shying away from active involvement in life as the struggle hurts too much. To break out of this unhappy state they need to feel empowered again and to believe that they can do something to improve their lot in life. The Wild Rose remedy offers that spark of vitality needed to dissolve away feelings of apathy and enter a renewed phase of optimism and personal growth.

Wild Rose for Dogs: Canine behaviourists talk about a type of dog behaviour called 'learned helplessness' which is very similar to the way people feel when they have become weary of struggling against life's challenges. Dogs that have been exposed to chronic stress for too long can begin to 'shut down' emotionally: they may lose the will to survive, becoming passive and resigned to whatever happens. It's a frozen state where they have learned that they're quite helpless and there's no point in resisting. This state is often seen in dogs that have been abused or treated cruelly for a long time. Dogs that have fallen ill, or may be slowly dying, can also suffer from this state. Wild Rose is an important Bach remedy for such dogs, as it helps to give them the strength to rekindle an interest in surviving and carrying on. One of its primary uses is in helping rescue dogs, who may have often suffered the kind of hardships that have made them 'shut down' emotionally. It can also be very supportive to elderly, sick or convalescing dogs. It works well together with remedies like Gorse, Oak, Olive and Gentian in helping to restore vitality to a depleted system. However, please remember that these are not medicines in their own right, and should not solely be relied upon if veterinary care is needed.

Veterinary associates of the Society for Animal Flower Essence Research have found that Wild Rose can be effective in helping injured wild animals, such as birds and rabbits, to survive the stresses of anaesthetic and operations. Very often these animals die on the operating table or soon after, not necessarily because of the injuries they've suffered but because the stress of being brought into a completely alien environment and handled by people is too much for them. This helps to give an idea of the potential of this remedy.

MUSTARD*

Latin name:	Sinapis arvensis
Dr Bach's words:	'Those who are liable to times of gloom, or even despair, as though a cold dark cloud overshadowed them and hid the light and the joy of life… under these conditions it's almost impossible to appear happy or cheerful'
Keynotes:	**Depression and gloom**
Goal of therapy:	**Optimism, light and joyfulness**

Mustard for People: Mustard's role is in helping with states of emotional gloom and dejection. A negative Mustard state can seem to descend like a black cloud, as though from nowhere, bringing a dark mood of depression that often can't be rationalised or explained. People sinking into this unhappy state of mind often lose all sense of joy and incentive, shrinking away from life and other people and lacking any mental energy to try to get back on their feet again. Mustard has been found to restore this incentive and help bring a little light back into their lives.

The Mustard state is quite closely related to the Wild Rose state, and the two remedies can work very well together if the person is suffering a feeling of apathy and resignation with no will to fight against their problems. It can also be very effective together with Olive, if the lack of mental energy and sense of prostration have come on due to energy depletion, for instance after a period of overwork or illness.

Mustard for Dogs: Dogs can also sometimes fall into states of depression and although it often seems to happen for no apparent reason in humans, there's usually a clear reason for this emotional state in a dog. Causes can be too much stress, loss of a friend, change in circumstances such as being forced to leave a place that offers comfort and security, illness or a feeling of insecurity in old age. In any of these situations there can be a loss of joy in life and a reduction in motivation for the dog. Mustard, perhaps in conjunction with other indicated remedies depending on the situation – for instance Impatiens or Agrimony for stress, Walnut for unsettling changes, Honeysuckle for loss, Wild Rose for emotional 'shutdown' – can help to restore a happier state in the same way it can in humans.

If a dog has suddenly become depressed, isn't interested in food, and seems to be very listless, it's advisable to have his physical health checked by the vet. If the dog requires medical treatment, Mustard is just one Bach remedy that can be used to help him to recover; in fact as Dr Bach observed, helping the emotions may be a very important part of the dog's overall treatment.

SWEET CHESTNUT*

Latin name:	Castanea sativa
Dr Bach's words:	'For those moments which happen to some people when the anguish is so great as to seem to be unbearable… when the mind or body feels as if it had borne to the uttermost limit of its endurance, when it seems there is nothing but destruction and annihilation left to face'
Keynotes:	**Despair and faithlessness**
Goal of therapy:	**Hope and endurance**

Sweet Chestnut for People: Sweet Chestnut deals with a very dark, grim state of mind, perhaps the darkest that a person can experience. People in need of this remedy are plagued by terrible emotional suffering and morbid, bitter feelings from which they can't escape. This can happen during harrowing times such as the loss of a loved one, or in very painful and severe diseases where there is a dark and pressing fear of death. A Sweet Chestnut state can also be the result of an existential crisis, where the sufferer has driven him or herself into a nihilistic depression by dwelling too much on the unanswerable questions of the human condition. For many, the idea that there is no meaning or purpose to life is too much to bear. This search for an elusive Truth has tormented humanity for thousands of years, and on a personal level this has created suffering and depression; on a global level it has given birth to religion which in turn has created division, hatred and war.

Sweet Chestnut helps to promote greater endurance, and a renewed sense of hope. Therapists often use it alongside Mustard for states of depression, and also in conjunction with Gorse and Star of Bethlehem. It can help to lighten states of extreme agony and help people get through the darkest experiences of their lives.

Sweet Chestnut for Dogs: Luckily for dogs, they don't have the capacity of humans to fall into states of existential crisis or depression associated with dark thoughts and ideas. They don't need to search for meaning in life, or understand 'what it's all about'. Dogs are free from the multiple human neuroses. They don't dwell on morbid ideas or begin to hate themselves. Their minds are a much clearer, simpler, and in many ways healthier place than ours. However, as sensitive and intelligent animals they are still capable of falling into very sad and anguished states of mind if they are sick, or left alone and abandoned, or suffering terrible neglect or stress. This is where Sweet Chestnut can be used to help them. A dog in need of this remedy may have experienced terrible hardships such as abandonment, cruelty or starvation. In other situations, dogs may have lost a beloved owner or companion and be in a state of extreme anxiety over this. Dogs that have suffered a great deal of physical hardship – and are weakened as a result – may need Sweet Chestnut and other remedies to help them recuperate and regain their strength and health. As in human therapy, remedies that may be chosen to work alongside Sweet Chestnut for dogs include Star of Bethlehem (extremely important in helping rescued or previously maltreated dogs), Gorse, Mustard, Wild Rose and Oak.

'RESCUE REMEDY'/5-FLOWER FORMULA*

Keynotes: **All-round emergency and crisis formula**

Goal of therapy: **To relax, calm, soothe and support**

Dr Bach designed only one ready-made combination remedy during his career. It's a mixture of Cherry Plum, Rock Rose, Impatiens, Clematis, and Star of Bethlehem. This classic formula is probably the best known of all Dr Bach's remedies, and for many people it's their first contact with this system of therapy. Quite often, you may meet someone who has never heard of Dr Bach or his work, but who has often used this famous combination remedy and trusts its efficacy. Many people use this remedy for general nerves, if they have to take an exam, if they have to go to the dentist, have to travel by plane, if they have had an argument and need to soothe their nerves, or if they have had a hard day at work.

The simple idea of this combination remedy is to provide fast-acting relief in any acute, urgent, pressing situation. There may be no time to plan a treatment program or to choose remedies for the individual. The emergency combination is the 'first aid kit' of the Bach remedies, ready for instant use in a wide variety of scenarios.

Because there are various different companies producing versions of Dr Bach's remedies, there are a variety of replicas of the classic combination formula available. In Britain, the original name 'Rescue Remedy' is retained by Nelsons, while Ainsworths homeopathic pharmacy produces their version named 'Recovery Remedy'. While these are perfectly effective and able to deliver wonderful results, the authors favour the version produced by Healing Herbs Ltd, called 'Five-Flower Formula'.

Whatever version of the original formula is used, it's a very effective aid for a wide variety of problems suffered by dogs. It can be used as a general anti-stress or calming remedy in all kinds of situations, and is a good thing to have around just in case of an accident or frightening event. If a dog is injured or suddenly falls sick and you are waiting for the vet to arrive or transporting the dog to the surgery, the remedy can be rubbed onto the gums or applied to the skin anywhere you can feel a pulse. The energy stored in the liquid will quickly find its way into the dog's system. For more information on methods of administering this and any other Bach remedy, see the chapter on *Practicalities of Giving Bach Remedies to Dogs*.

The various versions of the Rescue combination are also available in cream form, allowing some very interesting applications. Rescue or Five-Flower cream can be used as a safe all-round treatment for all kinds of skin problems, minor wounds, burns and aches. One of the most astounding cases the authors have come across with this cream wasn't a dog, but a pet bird that was flying around the owner's kitchen and accidentally landed in a pot of boiling soup that the owner was preparing for dinner! The bird's feet and legs were very badly scalded, with bleeding blisters and raw flesh. The vet didn't know what to do, and the bird was in such a bad condition that the devastated owner considered having him put to sleep to end his suffering. It was recommended that the owner tried applying some of the Healing Herbs 5-Flower Cream. Within **only one day** the healing of the bird's feet and legs had started, and after just a few days the bird was completely back to normal, showing no traces whatsoever of the incident.

There have been many, many cases of Rescue Remedy or 5-Flower Formula helping with emergency situations, acute fears, shock and trauma. However, because it's a generalised combination and isn't designed to take individual cases into account, you can create a much more flexible and individualised system of therapy by learning about the individual remedies and using them with skill and thought. While an effective combination remedy like this is a great thing to have in your pocket or at home 'just in case', the true satisfaction in using Bach remedies is to be able to choose from the whole range of remedies and become really familiar with the system.

Chapter Four

Bach Flower Remedies in Specific Areas of Canine Care

In this section we take a more detailed look into some specific types of problems and situations affecting dogs and their owners, and the role of Bach flower remedies in helping them.

Adolescence

Adolescence in dogs usually starts at around six months and may last up to the age of eighteen months, depending on the breed of dog. This is a time when dogs often become rather unruly and hard to handle, when many owners give up on them and find them a new home. For the dog it's a period of discovery, developing maturity and rebellion, much like the teen years of a human. Your dog may not be so willing to listen to you as he was in puppyhood, and he may appear more interested in the world around him than he is in you. Accept this as normal and be patient with him as the phase works itself out. Continue with your training, a little each day, and always make sure to end on a good note, even if it means you've only done five minutes.

Adolescence is obviously linked to the onset of sexual maturity, and both males and females will undergo fluctuations of hormone levels with quite noticeable changes in mood and behaviour. This is also quite normal as long as it's within reasonable limits – consult your vet if in any doubt.

Bach flower remedies to help:

- **Chestnut Bud:** For impulsiveness, youthful over-exuberance and tending not to absorb the lessons of training and discipline; dogs that may seem a bit 'scatty' and even stupid, making the same mistakes over and over again.

- **Vine:** This remedy is very useful for adolescence and young adulthood, dealing with impulsiveness and the tendency towards rebelliousness.

- **Walnut and Scleranthus:** These will both help to deal with changing hormonal levels as the dog grows up, and with temperament fluctuation (especially in bitches).

- **Impatiens:** This is more for the owner than the dog! Adolescent dogs will frequently try our patience to the limit; however we should not lose our temper with them as we stand to undo all the good work we have done so far. This remedy helps us to remain calm and not get annoyed.

Attention-seeking

This is another common problem that plagues dog owners. It can become a nightmare when your dog just will not leave you alone, or will not allow you to leave him alone.

Attention–seeking is really about control. Dogs are very good at getting our attention, and they have many ways of making sure they get it whenever they want it. Dogs are wonderful animals but they are also very clever opportunists! For them, your attention is a sign of their importance within the pack. By giving attention to a dog whenever he asks for it, you are giving out clear signals to the dog that he's a very high ranking wolf, and perhaps even higher ranking than you!

It often begins with us feeling flattered when our puppy or new dog starts coming over to us to 'say hello' in the form of a lick or a nudge, as we sit reading or watching TV. We will automatically respond with a pat on the head and a 'good dog', and maybe sometimes a treat too! In the dog's mind, the way to get affection and treats is to come up and just ask for them – it works every time! Before we know it, the dog is getting more and more insistent and constantly interrupting us for attention. Furthermore, as the situation escalates, many dogs start to dislike it when your attention is paid to anyone or anything else. Examples are the telephone, the TV, books and newspapers, other people, especially visitors. To get attention, dogs may whinge, bark, scratch at your leg, place a paw on you, stare pathetically at you, press themselves up against you, or even – larger breeds find this easier – reverse into you and sit on your knee. This is a great party trick that is all too often encouraged by the laughter of visitors.

There are times, of course, when your dog may have a very valid reason for trying to get your attention. He may be hungry, thirsty, or want to relieve himself. Sometimes it's hard, especially with very young dogs or old dogs that may be somewhat incontinent, to know when crying at 3 a.m. is attention seeking or an urgent cry to go out to urinate. Make sure such needs are attended to before concluding that the behaviour is attention-seeking.

An important way of preventing attention-seeking behaviour is to *stop giving your dog attention on demand*. This isn't to say that you should not show him affection. What you should do when he comes up to you is ignore him, then about fifteen minutes later, making sure he has totally given up trying to get your attention, call him over and make a big fuss of him. What you are doing here is taking control back from the dog. He no longer decides when he gets the attention – you decide. It's very important to have lots of contact with your dog, but this contact should be always on your terms. You decide when it starts and when it ends. This way, YOU are the leader of the pack, not the dog.

If you have a problem with an attention-seeking dog and you decide to start ignoring him and controlling the situation by making the first moves as a rule, you may find the dog resisting you and perhaps even sulking. Barking dogs may bark louder and longer, whining dogs will wail really loudly, and staring dogs will bore into you with laser-beam eyes. The reason is that they suddenly find their method for getting your attention is no longer working, and so they are 'Turning up the volume'.

How do we deal with this situation? The answer is that you must ignore the dog's attempt to gain attention. Here are the golden rules:

1. Do NOT look at the dog while he's trying to make eye contact with you

2. Do NOT speak or shout at the dog when he's looking for attention. Even a scolding constitutes attention!

3. Do NOT touch the dog when he tries to make physical contact as a way of getting attention. Move away without saying anything. Act as though the dog simply weren't there.

These will be extremely powerful signals that the dog will understand clearly. What they tell the dog is that his attempts to gain control over you aren't working any more. Sooner or later, depending on how tenacious he is, the dog will eventually give up his quest for attention-seeking.

The fourth golden rule is this: Do NOT give in! Once you have started this process, you MUST persevere. Give in, and you're in trouble. The dog will have learned that he CAN get your attention and CAN control you, by using certain techniques. This will be very hard to cure, as the dog will have won an important battle of wits against you. He has become your leader!

Luckily, Bach remedies come to the rescue to help with this common problem: Flower remedies can also help with this transition.

Bach flower remedies to help:

- **Chicory:** This helps to reduce the dog's strong desire to gain your attention. Remember, though, that this is a natural behaviour for the dog and no remedy can completely stop it.

- **Heather:** This would be helpful for reducing a dog's cloying attention-seeking ways, especially if he's very vocal with it.

- **Willow:** If the dog appears resentful and moody.

- **Vine:** To help negate the dog's controlling behaviour

For the owner, Impatiens can help to reduce the stress of having to wait while the dog's method of attention-grabbing diminishes. If you have allowed the situation to become extreme, the constant barking and howling can drive you crazy. If necessary, try Impatiens together with Cherry Plum and Holly to control your temper and resist the temptation to yell at the dog. Remember, yelling will solve nothing. It may be seen by the dog as the attention it wants, or it might also stress and confuse the dog. Another potentially useful remedy to help the owner in this situation is Centaury. Centaury is the remedy that helps you to assert your willpower, to say NO and to be firm and determined.

Lastly, some people develop a need for Pine during this process. Owners often feel guilty about ignoring their dog, and in fact this is one of the reasons why training programmes sometimes break down. There's often someone in the family (usually someone on the outside who doesn't have to put up with the dog all the time) who thinks the new regime is cruel or unfair. Don't listen to them, because that is not the case – in fact, taking these gentle steps to solve the problem is a blessing to the dog. Most attention-seeking dogs live in a high state of stress. The Pine remedy helps to alleviate the sense of guilt and helps you understand when guilt is unfounded.

Bereavement

A dog can feel severe grief at the death of an owner or of another animal that it has bonded with. As very social animals, dogs invest a great deal emotionally into their companions and can feel very lost when suddenly left alone. For a dog, it doesn't really make any difference whether their owner/companion is actually dead or simply not there any more. Dogs suddenly taken away from a stable environment where they were happy can feel as though their companions had suddenly all 'died'. What matters is the fact that the dog is left feeling alone, vulnerable and unprotected. This creates enormous stress that can bring about a serious shutdown the dog's emotions. They may fall into severe depression, stop eating, and even die. When we talk about humans dying 'of a broken heart', this is exactly what can happen to dogs.

Dogs are also very affected by the grief of humans when someone dies. This could be the death of a relative, friend, or of another animal. When the dog sees its leaders and companions acting in a distraught manner, perhaps crying, acting oddly, or feeling down and sad, this all creates stress in the dog's mind. The dog's sense of social security is weakened. What's happening to the pack? Dogs don't like it when the pack is acting oddly. They are emotionally tied to their pack: when everyone's happy, dogs are happy. But when everyone is upset, the dog is stressed and vulnerable.

Bach flower remedies to help:

- **Star of Bethlehem:** To help dogs recover from the shock of grief and loss.

- **Gorse:** Can help to brighten the emotional state of a dog that is very downcast, broken-hearted or giving up the will to live.

- **Sweet Chestnut:** Similar to Gorse, to help bring some light into a very dark and bleak outlook.

- **Wild Rose:** For dogs that have fallen into a resigned state of apathy where they no longer care about anything.

- **Honeysuckle:** Can help a dog to recover emotionally from the loss of old friends and companions.

- **Walnut:** Helps the dog to adapt to major changes in its life, giving strength and resilience to move on from the event and become happy again. This remedy also helps to protect the dog from feeling too badly affected by the negative feelings of others around, for instance in the case of a death in the family where the dog witnesses the sadness of its owners.

Humans should also consider using Bach remedies at a time when your pet is very sick and has to be put to sleep by the vet, to help you and the dog stay calm and composed during this difficult time. People bond closely with their dogs and their passing creates a lot of emotional pain. Old people, who may have nobody else for company, can sometimes go into decline after losing a pet, and it isn't unknown for them to die soon after the pet. Bach remedies such as Star of Bethlehem, Gorse, Sweet Chestnut, Wild Rose and Mustard could help to prevent this from happening.

Another reason for trying to stay composed during this time is our responsibility to other animals in the household. Remaining dogs may feel upset by the sudden loss of their companion, but their stress and sadness will be compounded by seeing the pack in turmoil. In some cases, this may even account for the greater part of the emotional stress they feel at the time of the dog's death.

We also need to remain calm around a dog who is dying or soon to be put to sleep. Dogs are very sensitive to our feelings and the emotional atmosphere, and if you allow the dog to sense that you are terribly upset and heartbroken, this could make his last few hours a time of stress and fear. If we can act calmly and peacefully, this will help the dog to leave this life in a more relaxed and reassured state of mind. This is a tribute of respect for the feelings of a loved animal that will soon no longer be with us. So for all these reasons it's important to use Bach remedies at a time of pet loss.

Car travel problems

There are many different problems that can occur with dogs in cars. These are usually stress related, especially if the dog hasn't been taught to be relaxed in the car or if the dog has had some kind of negative experience associated with travelling.

If your dog is afraid of going in the car, try some of the following ideas to help desensitise it:

1. Leave the back of the car open when parked in your driveway, letting your dog spend some time in it on his own with a bone, snack or toy to chew. Note: leave the car open, and never keep a dog inside a car for too long in hot weather!

2. When the dog is comfortable being inside the car, try taking him on 'mock' trips by driving a short distance (e.g. to the bottom of the road and back) and then giving him a pleasurable reward such as a walk or a game.

3. Build this up until your dog actively looks forward to going places in the car.

Bach flower remedies to help:

- **Mimulus:** For general fears and anxieties; dogs that whine and tremble in the car, and so on.

- **Rock Rose:** For dogs whose fears borders more on terror, with panicky behaviour and perhaps scrabbling to get out. **Cherry Plum** could help here too.

- **Star of Bethlehem:** If fears and travelling problems have come about because of a past trauma associated with the car, e.g. an accident, using this remedy will help release the after-effects and the memory of the incident. (See Jacques' case, later in the book)

- **Rescue remedy:** As the three remedies above, Rock Rose, Mimulus and Star of Bethlehem, are all to be found within the classic combination formula, you could very easily use this instead for its effective calming outcome.

- **Scleranthus:** A fairly common problem is dogs vomiting in moving cars. Scleranthus is reported to be quite effective for cases of motion sickness and is one of the occasional examples of Bach remedies working more on the physical level.

Emergency situations

Urgent or emergency situations in a dog's life may include many types of things, including:

- Being attacked by another dog
- Suffering an accident
- Experiencing a severe fright
- Requiring urgent medical treatment and becoming highly stressed

Each situation will have to be dealt with in its own way, but whatever the case Bach remedies can be used to help in two main ways:

1. To assist with the immediate problem and its psychological effect, for instance fear, terror, panic, distress, out of control behaviour

2. To assist with the after-effects of the experience, helping to ensure that it doesn't remain lodged in the dog's psyche as a traumatic memory that could create all kinds of anxiety-related problems in the future.

Bach flower remedies to help:

- **Star of Bethlehem:** Star of Bethlehem is always the first Bach remedy we should think of when there has been any kind of traumatic situation, whether it's a recent happening or something that happened long ago. The remedy plays a crucial dual role in trauma management, having the unique ability not only to help an immediate problem but also to help prevent a recent traumatic incident from becoming a problem in the future. It's also a good idea for humans to take some Star of Bethlehem if they're involved in an accident or emergency situation involving their dog. The remedy is one of the key ingredients in:

- **Rescue Remedy/5 Flower Formula:** This classic combination remedy is intended for all emergency situations, such as deep shock following accident or injury, collapse, severe frights, etc. As well as the vitally important Star of Bethlehem this combination contains Rock Rose, Cherry Plum and Impatiens, all potentially capable in their different ways of significantly reducing the psychological distress of a traumatic or emergency incident.

- **Wild Rose, Gorse, Mustard, Gentian, Olive:** These would be used in the aftermath of the emergency, if the dog has lost interest in life and has become listless and apathetic. You should obviously have the dog regularly checked by the vet to ensure this is not a medical problem.

Fear and anxiety

We have all experienced fear and anxiety and therefore we can understand subjectively, without having to go into dog psychology, how deeply fear can affect our dogs.

Fear comes in many different shapes and sizes. There are the frights that accompany traumatic events such as being attacked by another dog, or being in an accident. Long-term fearfulness may result from these incidents. Training and behavioural work can help, but sometimes do not resolve the problem fully. Flower remedies can get to the root of the matter, repairing at an energy level the emotional damage that is causing the fear in the first place.

Bach flower remedies to help:

- **Mimulus:** This remedy addresses everyday, ongoing mild fears and anxieties. It isn't generally used for acute panic or very extreme fear or terror. People and animals that have developed mild phobias will often benefit from Mimulus. Larch could also be included here as it addresses lack of confidence.

- **Rock Rose:** Rock Rose is used for very extreme kinds of fear, terror or panic. It's quite easy to tell the level of fear in a dog. A very scared dog will tremble, cower, perhaps roll over in submission, perhaps wet itself, or just freeze to a standstill in absolute terror as it just gives in to imminent death. In this type of case Rock Rose is called for, perhaps along with Star of Bethlehem.

- **Five Flower Formula/Rescue Remedy:** This combination will be of great value in helping to calm acute states of fear, and is always worth carrying in your pocket 'just in case'.

- **Star of Bethlehem:** If you think that a fear or anxiety might have roots in a past traumatic incident or anything that the dog may have experienced before you knew him, Star of Bethlehem can be used to help with the emotional scars from the past that have not healed. Giving this remedy together with remedies for the present fear can be very effective.

One of the problems with fear in dogs is that it's very easy to accidentally reinforce the anxiety by rewarding it. For instance, if a dog gets a fright and comes running back to you as its leader, you may think the best response is to give the dog a cuddle and some reassuring words. In fact, this is likely to have the opposite effect, and actually reinforce the fear by rewarding the behaviour!

The best thing to do in such an instance is to *ignore the dog completely.* Act as coolly as possible, turn away and pretend to be doing something else. This may seem somewhat counter-intuitive, but it makes perfect sense in dog terms. It's giving the dog the powerful signal that the pack leader isn't worried about whatever it was that frightened it. If the leader isn't worried, then the dog will begin to think there's nothing to worry about at all. Ignoring the dog is doing three positive things:

1. Reinforcing your position as his leader

2. Reassuring the dog without rewarding the fear

3. Helping to prevent further anxiety as well as attention-seeking problems

Hyperactivity

The cause of hyperactivity is very likely due to dietary matters, lack of exercise leading to boredom, or a lack of control on the part of the owner. Many types of 'hyperactive' behaviour can be a dog's way of expressing a stressed state of mind. If a dog has had good basic training, has a healthy rapport with its owner, doesn't suffer from mental stress, gets adequate exercise, plenty of mental stimulation and a proper diet, it will tend not to act hyperactively.

Before you get a dog, consider your own lifestyle and how it will fit in with the requirements of different sizes and breeds of dog. A sheep-herding type dog, bred for running over wide spaces in the great outdoors, will often get bored and become a problem in a small flat in the city.

The following Bach remedies can help in some cases, but it's most important to isolate and rectify the real cause of this much misunderstood problem. If the remedies don't help or only help a little, this simply means that you will need to look deeper to see what is causing the problem.

Bach flower remedies to help:

- **Vervain:** May help for excessive exuberance and the tendency to use up too much energy.

- **Chestnut Bud:** For youthful impulsiveness, to help calm and mellow the dog's urge to run around like a mad thing.

- **Impatiens:** May help to calm nervous and highly strung animals that rush around. Impatiens can be very effective at helping to reduce stress and relax a dog.

- **Five Flower Formula/Rescue Remedy:** A general calming remedy

Old age

Aging is a natural process that comes to us all, the gradual and inevitable deterioration of the organism that has acted as host and vehicle to the vital spark that is 'us'. Just like humans, when dogs reach a certain age they experience changes in both body and mind. Just when old age begins to show in a dog depends on various factors:

- General state of health: a healthier dog will resist the symptoms of aging for longer.

- Emotional stability: likewise, a happy dog will tend go on for much longer before old age begins to take its toll.

- Breed: thanks to our random genetic experimentation on the original DNA of the wolf, many breeds live relatively short lives. Breeds such as the Jack Russell terrier tend to be sturdy and long-lived, while others such as the Scottish deerhound often barely make it to the age of seven.

Problems that commonly afflict the elderly dog include:

- Loss of confidence due to hierarchy shift: in any multi-dog household the dogs are always conscious of their internal politics. It's a natural consequence of aging that a dog that's always held a leadership position relative to the other dog or dogs in its group will, at a certain stage, begin to lose its grip on that position. If there's another dog waiting in line to take up that role, signs that the leader is growing older and slower may be his cue to challenge for leadership. This is perfectly normal behaviour, intended to keep the pack strong. However this loss of status can have an adverse impact on the old dog, damaging his general confidence.

- Fears and insecurity: older dogs often become fearful, anxious or confused. This can happen after a traumatic incident, such as an operation – which older dogs may have to go through as their health weakens – or a frightening incident. Older dogs sometimes suffer from night-time fears. As a result of anxiety, these 'old timers' may start to go downhill physically, with a loss of general tone and possibly a loss of resistance to illness.

- Sense of vulnerability as physical power diminishes: the weakening of physical powers can have an effect on the dog's mind, making this once strong and self-assured animal begin to feel less confident and more vulnerable. Sometimes, the onset of fears and anxiety is a sign of developing illness, so if an older dog displays an uncharacteristic loss of confidence, it's important to have him checked over by the vet, just in case.

Bach flower remedies to help:

- **Mimulus, Larch and Aspen:** To help with fears and loss of confidence associated with aging. Aspen may be especially helpful to reduce anxiety caused by failing health, although it shouldn't be seen as a substitute for veterinary attention.

- **Star of Bethlehem:** Good to consider in case a frightening experience has been traumatic enough to affect the dog's confidence.

- **Oak, Gentian and Olive:** These remedies can all help to maintain the older dog's energy and zest for living. All three have a potential use to help the dog through periods of illness, when vital energy may dip.

- **Honeysuckle:** This remedy often helps older dogs whose companions have died, resulting in a sense of loneliness and insecurity. See the above section on Bereavement.

- **Walnut:** Can help the older dog adapt to changes that come in the later stages of life, such as hierarchy shifts that result from his loss of power. Walnut may also help in adapting to reduced physical powers, such as the weakening of agility and stamina.

- **Mustard, Wild Rose and Gorse:** To offer support through times of dejection and reduced joy of life, and to help regenerate the will to go on. However, please bear in mind the following important note:

Note: Eventually, the dog is going to reach the end of the line. Bach remedies can do a great deal to promote a happy life for him while he is still able to enjoy it. However, sooner or later owners of elderly dogs will have to face the decision whether or not it's in the dog's best interests to prolong his life. It would be cruel and pointless to try to depend on Bach remedies to keep a dog going if he is suffering. At that point we need to take responsibility to do the right thing if necessary. If we think it best to end the dog's suffering, we need to act quickly and decisively for his sake. Bach remedies can help us with that painful and difficult process – please see the section on pet bereavement in the next chapter.

Puppyhood

Puppies and young dogs can benefit from Bach remedies in a number of ways. Sometimes, remedies may be needed to help with problems that have arisen – these could include just about any of the problems Bach remedies are needed for generally, for instance: fears, trauma, emergencies. Another important role for Bach remedies in helping dogs at this delicate, formative time of their lives is to help shape their personalities so they will be grow up to be psychologically strong, confident and well-rounded adults. Lessons learned and mental pathways developed at this early age will set the dog up for life, and so it's crucial to guide the process carefully and sensibly.

Bringing home a new puppy for the first time, we should be aware of how bewildered the little creature may be feeling. Unless born into your household, he will have just been parted from his mother and littermates, moved from the only place he's ever known to a strange and unfamiliar environment full of unknown creatures, sounds and smells. While some pups seem to settle in without difficulty, others may experience considerable emotional turmoil at this time. Make sure the pup has plenty of rest in a secure place and isn't disturbed. Inquisitive and excited children should be told firmly to leave him alone until he settles. Children often exhaust a puppy by wanting to play with him all the time, so parents should keep their eyes open for this.

Socialisation is a vitally important part of the puppy's early formation. He needs to be gently introduced to a wide variety of experiences early on, in order to equip him with the mental 'software' to deal with any situation as he grows up. It's especially important to socialise the dog with people, adults and children, as well as other dogs. See the section on *Socialisation* in the following pages.

Formal training is something to leave until a little later in the dog's life, but right from the start it's important to encourage him to learn positive lessons. He needs to learn many things: toilet training, good manners, not to mouth or bite people, and to begin to recognise certain signals and commands. This is a period of intense learning for the dog, and the process needs to be shaped properly in order to ensure his development into a happy and well-rounded adult.

Bach remedies to help:

- **Mimulus and Larch:** These are important in helping to form a secure and confident personality in the puppy from the start. There's no harm in giving drops to the pup even if he isn't necessarily showing signs of anxiety: reducing even the smallest feelings of nervousness will help at this stage to prevent future temperament problems.

- **Cerato:** Along with Larch, this remedy can help the puppy to form a strong, confident outlook. Together with sensible training – e.g. not allowing the pup to become emotionally dependent on you – the remedy helps to foster a well-balanced and healthily independent spirit.

- **Walnut:** Sudden changes, such as being whisked away from everything he's known to find himself in an alien environment, can be unsettling. Walnut helps to strengthen the puppy's emotional resistance and allow him to adapt comfortably and confidently. Walnut also helps in socialisation, to help the young dog deal with all the new sights, sounds and places.

- **Elm:** This is an important remedy to help reduce the 'sensory overload' the pup may experience when coming into his new home for the first time, and then, later on, during the crucial socialisation process.

- **Chestnut Bud:** Helps a developing mind to form positive associations and learn important lessons for life. The remedy fosters a young dog's intelligence, often appearing to sharpen cognitive skills and encourage quick logical thinking. An important early learning remedy.

Recuperation from illness

It's often forgotten that Dr Bach's main initial reason for developing the flower remedies was actually his interest in psychoneuroimmunology – the study of how the emotions affect physical health. Helping all living creatures to cope with illness is an important part of Bach flower therapy, even though the remedies are not themselves intended to cure diseases.

Bach remedies to help:

In fact, it's quite true to say that just about all 38 remedies can, in their separate ways, help to keep a dog healthy by generally promoting emotional happiness, confidence and vitality throughout his life. A happy dog will generally tend to be less prone to illness in the first place than a stressed or unhappy dog, and better equipped to deal with it if it should strike. However, if and when a dog falls ill for any reason, is injured or has to have an operation, there are certain key remedies that are often indicated to help him through this time and help promote healthy healing.

- **Gorse and Wild Rose:** To help against sinking spirits, despondency and loss of the will to go on.

- **Star of Bethlehem:** To help protect against the damaging, traumatic impact of operations or other unpleasant experiences the dog may have to endure during illness.

- **Aspen:** To help the dog deal with unconscious fears and feelings of vulnerability associated with illness.

- **Impatiens:** To help the dog deal with stress and mental tension. Dogs that have to be still and rested for a while, e.g. while a leg is in plaster or a wound is healing, can be helped to be more relaxed and patient.

- **Gentian, Hornbeam and Olive:** To help keep the vital energy maintained during illness, and help to promote a more positive recovery.

Rescue dogs

It's a very sad fact that many dogs are treated badly by people, ranging from neglect to active cruelty. There are many ways that people are cruel to dogs: by not feeding them, by making them suffer from terrible stress, and by physically harming them. Some very cruel people harm dogs deliberately, for fun. In Britain (and other countries) dogs are also bred under terrible conditions so that the puppies can be sold for big profits. This is called 'puppy farming' and it often involves a great deal of suffering to the dogs. The dogs are often kept in filthy conditions, in the dark, and underfed. Bitches that are no longer able to breed are often abandoned or killed. Dogs that survive this experience are often very traumatised, afraid of people, or have turned aggressive. Some are completely undersocialised with people and even with other dogs. Some have never been inside a human home and are very fearful of coming into the house.

Many countries have dog rescue organisations that care for the victims of abuse and cruelty. They deal with:

- Dogs that have been taken away from unsuitable owners

- Dogs that have been abandoned because the people did not want to give them food or medical care

- Dogs whose owners could not cope with their behaviour or could not afford to keep them

- Dogs whose owners have died and relatives rejected the animal

- Dogs that have run away from home

The work of these rescue centres and animal welfare organisations is to take the dogs in, give them the appropriate care, and try if possible to rehome them with caring new owners in a suitable environment. This work can be very upsetting, as so many dogs are emotionally traumatised or physically so damaged that there is little hope for them. They often have severe behaviour problems. These dogs are called 'rescue' dogs because they have literally been rescued from situations and environments that were unsuitable or harmful.

Taking in a rescue dog is a challenge, similar to fostering a child from a difficult background such as a war orphan. Ideally, someone who takes in a rescue dog should have good knowledge of dogs – it may be unwise to have a rescue as your first dog. Giving the dog lots of care and love is important but even this on its own is often not enough to help a dog with emotional problems. However, Bach flower remedies can often help with many of the problems of traumatised or abused dogs.

Bach remedies to help:

- **Star of Bethlehem:** This is one of the most important remedies for all animals with a difficult past. One of the problems with rescue dogs is that we often don't know what the dog has been through. We can get clues from his behaviour; for instance, if you raise your arm to take a book off the shelf or to brush your hair and the dog immediately cringes and goes into a submissive body posture, you know someone may have beaten that dog. Star of Bethlehem can be given to ANY rescue dog 'just in case' of past maltreatment and trauma. It's a very deep-acting and fundamental remedy.

- **Mimulus and Rock Rose:** Most problems with rescue dogs are due to fear. Experience of life often has taught them to be fearful of many things, especially humans. It's very important to use these fear remedies for such a dog. These remedies may have to be given to the dog for a long time, perhaps even forever in some cases. It may be that Mimulus or Rock Rose only partially help to reduce the fear of a rescue dog. This is often because they are only addressing the 'outer layer' of the problem, the fears themselves. If the fears are caused by a deeper problem, such as past traumas experienced by the dog, Star of Bethlehem can be added to the dog's remedies to create a fuller effect.

- **Wild Rose, Gorse and Mustard:** These remedies can be needed for dogs that have fallen into depressed states as a result of long-term traumatic life experience. Star of Bethlehem will also serve in this role, but multiple remedies over a period of time will tend to have a better effect.

- **Holly, Willow, Beech and Water Violet:** In all their various ways, these remedies can often help to soften the attitude of a dog who has only ever known humans as persecutors and tormentors. It isn't recommended that anyone take on a rescue dog with aggression problems – sadly these are very often put to sleep. However, even a non-aggressive rescue can have a hardened and mistrustful attitude to humans, and we can't blame them for that. We may know we have the dog's best interests at heart, but the dog can only learn this slowly, over a period of time. It's up to us to show the dog that he can trust us. The role of the Bach remedies in this process is to gently work at the dog's emotions, allowing for that new trust to grow and develop.

Separation anxiety

This term refers to dogs that for one reason or another can't stand being left alone. Sometimes dogs that haven't been used to solitude are suddenly put into situations where they are alone for long periods: for instance when owners take a new job outside the home. Other examples occur when dogs have become too used to following their owners around the house and will not tolerate being left on their own, even for very short periods.

Problems such as excessive barking, howling, destructiveness (e.g. chewing scratching, digging) and fouling in the home may all occur with separation anxiety. Flower remedies can help, but the onus is also on the owner to bring up the dog in a way that he is used to being alone, for reasonable periods of time, and can cope with it. Some of the golden rules of preventing and solving this common problem are:

- *Don't* let the dog always follow you from room to room. This tends to create a problem of over-bonding where the dog is lacking in emotional independence.

- *Don't* make a big fuss of the dog when you leave the house – act casually and the dog will not think too much of it.

- *Always* keep dogs mentally and physically stimulated to prevent boredom.

Bach flower remedies to help:

- **Honeysuckle:** This is useful for many of the more 'straight-forward' cases of separation anxiety; where the dog is just 'feeling the blues' because of the owner's absence. He may express this by soulful howling. Honeysuckle is for states of 'I want things back to the way they were before' and so would be useful if the dog were pining for an owner who will not return, possibly who has died.

- **Gorse:** This would be called for in a dog that is truly despairing, close to grief, over the absence of a beloved owner. Again, when an owner has passed away, a dog may pine bitterly and sometimes even give up the will to live. Gorse is a great rebuilder of the vital force.

- **Walnut:** This remedy can help the dog to build up a sense of emotional independence, which is needed if he's to feel secure on his own.

- **Willow:** This can help the spoilt dominant type of dog that is actively resentful about being left alone.

- **Vine:** This can help to reduce the dog's urge to dominate and regard himself as the Alpha in the pack.

Socialisation

This is a very important part of any dog's training. Dogs have to be socialised from an early age with adults, children, other dogs and any animals they may encounter, and also with life in general. If a dog isn't properly socialised, he may grow up to be a fearful, unpredictable and sometimes aggressive animal. It's possible to socialise an older dog, but the earlier you start, the better. Many dog training books give useful tips on socialising your puppy or adult dog.

Flower remedies can help with the process of socialisation, by easing some of the blocks such as lack of confidence, fears, and vulnerability to too many bewildering outside impressions.

Bach flower remedies to help:

- **Chestnut Bud:** To help the dog process new information and to learn from the experience.

- **Mimulus and Larch:** These two remedies would be very useful to give to any young dog being introduced to the world, people and other animals for the first time.

- **Elm:** This can help the young dog not to feel overwhelmed by the huge number of new sense impressions he's experiencing when you take him out into the world for the first time. For a dog that has never seen crowds, traffic, and all the busy world that we take for granted, it can be very emotionally tiring and even stressful. The remedy helps the dog to process all this new information without becoming too overloaded. This will also help a lot to create a confident and happy dog in the future.

- **Walnut:** This can help to 'shield' the dog from too many confusing impressions from the outside and help (like Elm) to let the dog process all the sights, sounds, and smells without stress.

- **Water Violet:** Can help the dog to bond to his new owner, members of the household and other animals in the new pack, whether these be dogs, cats or other animals.

Chapter Five

Owners who need
Bach Remedies

So far in this book we've covered many ways that Bach flower remedies can help dogs by addressing many canine psychological, emotional and behavioural problems. However, helping the dogs themselves by giving them the benefit of these fascinating remedies isn't the whole story. Because our dogs' lives are so closely intertwined with ours, it's a sad fact that they don't just suffer from canine problems: they suffer our problems too!

When humans become stressed, tense, angry, sad, despondent – whatever the case may be – dogs will very often pick up on these emotions. They don't necessarily, as has sometimes been said, 'mirror' our emotions: for instance if you are angry about something, your dog doesn't respond by getting angry too. If he shows a response to your going about the house shouting and thumping the walls, it will be one of fear, anxiety and confusion. *What's going on? Is there something I should know? Is something wrong with my pack? Is my human angry at me? Is he going to shout at me or attack me?* Those might be some of the thoughts passing through his mind. You may notice dogs giving calming signals, such as licking their lips or blinking their eyes, as a means of trying to calm their distraught pack-mate. Usually, humans don't notice these signals, and go on stressing the dog. It may not be their fault that they're anxious, upset, angry, etc., but nonetheless they should try to calm down for their dog's sake if not for their own.

Bach remedies are a key therapy to help with this process of preventing what is known as 'sponge effect', the effect whereby a dog will literally soak up the negative energy that comes pouring off their stressed-out humans. Below are some examples of how different remedies can help.

Agrimony

The person needing this remedy often suffers from mental torment that they keep to themselves. They may be able to hide it from other people, but a dog that is very close to his owner may be able to pick up on it. As a result, dogs can become very depressed, lack vitality, and be more prone to illness.

Chicory

Chicory is a state of self-centredness. The person needing Chicory may get a dog to serve their ego as opposed to getting a dog they really care for. Many insecure people use animals to boost their own self-esteem, enjoying the attention they receive in return for constant titbits and snacks – essentially buying 'love' from the animal in order to feel better themselves, a kind of eating disorder by proxy. Many such owners render their dogs seriously overweight and unhealthy by this rather self-centred behaviour. Chicory owners also tend to create emotionally over-dependent dogs that are likely to suffer from separation anxiety problems when left alone. The lesson learned by taking Chicory is one of thoughtful, selfless service to others, and this is a very important attribute for a caring dog owner.

Vervain

The type of person needing Vervain may tend to be very active and always rushing about, or making a lot of noise. This may create a very hyper-active dog or one that is deprived of peace and rest. It would especially be a problem for young puppies, which need lots of sleep throughout the day. The Vervain person may be so over-the-top that a more submissive type of dog could be afraid of them and made nervous.

Centaury

The person needing Centaury often finds it very difficult to assert themselves. Part of having a healthy relationship with a dog is to be a kind and gentle, but firm and confident, leader. Someone who has problems being firm and decisive will always have trouble in a leadership role. They may create a very spoilt or dominant dog as they will find it very hard to say no. Many dogs will suffer from stress as a result, as forcing them to take the role of leader (every pack must have one!) may be more responsibility than they can handle.

Cerato

Like Centaury, the person needing Cerato lacks confidence. They are open to the suggestions of all self-appointed experts of whom there are many! This could be very dangerous. There was one case of a Cerato type of person who tied their dog up and beat him because a 'dog expert' had told them to do so. Also, the insecurities and fears of a Cerato type will tend to rub off on the dog, taking away the sense of a strong well-led pack and making him fearful and nervous. Pack animals need a confident leader.

Water Violet

The person needing Water Violet likes to keep a distance from others. Someone like this could create a very undersocialised dog which could potentially become fearful, or even fearfully aggressive. The Water Violet person often believes that they know best (the opposite of the Cerato person, who always believes someone else knows best!) and will never take anyone's suggestions on board, even if they really are experts!

Scleranthus

Scleranthus is the indecisive sort of person. They may have got a dog for the wrong reason. They can never decide what to do. They will tend to vacillate on training, never able to stick to a regime where constancy is required. Part of being a good owner is to create a steady balanced environment where a dog will feel secure. A person who is constantly changing their mind all the time will never be able to achieve this, and the effect on the dog will be very negative.

Gentian

People needing Gentian are very easily discouraged. This could cause problems if they bring a young dog into the home and things do not go according to plan. For example if a puppy is slow to be house-trained, the Gentian owner may become despondent and give up, saying: 'what's the point? I'll never be able to train him'. They may even decide to get rid of the puppy as they lack the dedication to overcome the small difficulties and challenges that come with dog ownership. If they allow themselves to get discouraged by the setbacks and problems of everyday life, they may become quite depressed and lacking in self-esteem. The dog will tend to pick up on these negative emotions and may also become very nervous and low in spirits, with resulting behaviour problems.

Rock rose

This type of person has a tendency to suffer from panic and sometimes very extreme fear. As a result, they may lack a great deal of confidence generally. A dog, being a pack animal, is going to notice this immediately, and his response may be one of great anxiety. If the dog should feel obliged to take on the obviously vacant role of pack leader, he may either become very dominant or very stressed by the responsibility – either of which will tend to cause its own problems.

Impatiens

These types of people want to run before they can walk! When dealing with young animals or animals in training the Impatiens type of person may often expect too much, too soon. If the dog doesn't respond immediately to lessons, the Impatiens type may become angry, shout at the dog or even punish him physically. This type of behaviour will cause a breakdown in the relationship between human and dog. The dog will become confused and perhaps stressed to the point of fearfulness. If the problem goes on long enough, with the dog forced to live with someone who intimidates him, the dog may eventually no longer trust people.

Clematis

People needing the Clematis remedy often lack interest in life. They tend to be dreamers and live in a world of their own. As a result, they may neglect their dog and not attend to his needs. They will often be unable to form a good bond with the dog. Clematis people may also be a bit too dreamy and far away to be of much use as a dog trainer! So their dog is likely to have been left badly untrained and possibly out of control. The remedy can help to bring such people back to earth and help them to attend to the neglected details of everyday life.

Mimulus

People needing Mimulus often suffer from niggling fears or are generally of a nervous or timid disposition. Again this will have an ongoing negative effect on their dog. The dog will feel insecure because he sees his pack has no strong leader and is like an army regiment without a commanding officer. This will force the dog to try to take on the leader's role himself. Just like the dog belonging to the Rock Rose owner, he may end up being very stressed and insecure, or he may rise to the position of leader and become very dominant, perhaps aggressive, possessive and controlling over resources such as people, territory and food.

Pet bereavement: when we lose a dog

One of the sad facts of having dogs is that they don't live very long compared to humans. The life span of many dogs is actually shortened because of humans' genetic manipulation of their original wild DNA: hardly any man-made dog breeds live as long as a wolf can live in the wild, and some breeds live tragically and absurdly short lives of as little as seven, even six, years.

But even if all dogs lived for twenty years or more, it would still mean that nearly every dog owner would experience the death of a loved pet dog at some stage. Every dog owner knows that the day will come when their beloved dog is no longer with them, yet when that day does arrive or approach, owners are often quite unprepared for it. Anxiety and hurt may be very considerable and the additional responsibility of having to make the decision to end the life of a suffering dog, adds more stress and pain.

In some countries such as Britain, there are helplines available for people needing emotional support after losing a dog. Helpline workers report that people can be so heartbroken at their dog's death that some of them feel suicidal. Many callers express to the counsellors that the dog's death has affected them more painfully than the death of a human friend or relative. Some people aren't comfortable about admitting this, breaking as it does our 'taboo' belief that human life has a greater value than animal life. However, if you feel this way it's nothing to be ashamed about: it just means that you loved your dog a great deal.

Bach flower remedies offer a highly effective and flexible means of helping people to cope with sadness and grief at the death of a pet dog. Factors to deal with may include:

1. The shock of hearing of the pet's death, finding him dead or seeing him killed, e.g. in a road accident.

2. The impact of being told by a vet, perhaps completely unexpectedly, that the pet's life is coming to an end or that he's suffering greatly and it would be the right thing to put him to sleep. In both these examples a very helpful remedy is *Star of Bethlehem,* which helps to reduce the impact of the shock. Many people use the *5-Flower Formula* in such instances and find that it really helps them.

3. The guilt and regret associated with having to have an animal put to sleep – sometimes with self-blame at perhaps not having kept a closer check on the pet's health or safety – can sometimes be great. There may also be mental torment over the sense of having neglected the pet's interests, perhaps at a time when other pressing issues to do with money/family/business etc. were presenting a distraction. Guilt and regret can also occur if the owner comes to believe that they may have acted too hastily, that something might have been done, that another vet might have been able to help, that the diagnosis/prognosis might have been incorrect, that they should have tried some other form of treatment, etc., etc. The negative effects of guilt and regret over past actions can be extremely damaging. The main Bach flower remedy to help with this is, of course, *Pine.*

4. The inability, whether through sentimentality, personal insecurity, indecisiveness or the belief that the dog 'will not forgive' them, to make the decision to have him put to sleep.

Bach flower remedies, especially *Scleranthus* (and maybe *Cerato*) can often help with this kind of indecision, vacillation, swaying over this option or that. The person's feelings of guilt may also be a large part of the motivation behind such procrastination. There is also the fear that many people have of being deprived of the warmth of a pet's companionship or of being left alone. This fear tells us something about the person's inner insecurities, and there may be remedies to help with that, for instance *Chicory* if the person is unwilling to let go of the comforting friendship even though the dog is suffering. Unfortunately, if the dog is very sick and suffering a lot, the end result of hesitation can only be more suffering for the animal. A surprising number of pet owners will keep sick animals alive in pain rather than face their responsibilities and/or fears. Then, when the dog finally dies or is found dead, the person will often have to face the strong pain of guilt and regret because they allowed this to happen.

5. The sense of separation and nostalgia after the death, which may be very prolonged and develop into severe depression in some cases. For these kinds of problems we have *Star of Bethlehem,* which is very important; *Gorse, Sweet Chestnut* and *Mustard* for feelings of despair and depression, and *Honeysuckle* for the feelings of painful nostalgia that prey on the mind. *Wild Rose* can be important is people have sunk into a state of apathy and have lost the will to get up and get on with life.

A real case of pet loss: Mary and Bill

Mary, 73, lost her dog Bill to old age. Mary and Bill had been sole companions for eight years, ever since the loss of her husband, Jack. Mary had never been alone. She had always gone out for walks with Bill, keeping herself fit and active. Now she seldom left the house. She lost interest in eating and could think and talk of nothing other than Bill, her times with him, his ways and habits: she would weep continually at the mention of his name. She additionally experienced a renewal of the pain she had undergone at the death of her husband, indicating that the grief over that loss had not been fully worked through. She appeared to lose colour and weight very fast. Her daughter Kate travelled to see her, very concerned that her mother's health might rapidly deteriorate. At first she pleaded with her mother to try and rise above her state;

then she would lose her temper and say: 'Look, if you don't snap out of this, you're going to fade away and die.' Mary replied that she didn't care, and in fact was looking forward to death as a means of becoming reunited with Jack and Bill. Kate's impression was that her mother was looking forward to that reunion happening as soon as possible – that she no longer wanted to live.

Kate approached a Bach flower therapist with regard to her mother's condition. It was agreed that the shock and grief might indeed spark a rapid physical decline. Mary was a fit and strong lady, and should have many years of active living ahead of her. Remedy selection was:

- Gorse for the general effects of grief and loss

- Star of Bethlehem for the shock to the system she had suffered and the stirring up of old hurt

- Gentian to help foster the courage to overcome this hard time and go forward

- Sweet Chestnut for her extreme sadness and black despair

- Wild Rose for her apathy and loss of will to live

- Honeysuckle for the tendency to dwell over the past

- Clematis for the dreamy state she had fallen into, losing her vital spark and spending her days in reverie about being reunited with her loved ones, not paying any heed to the loved ones still on this earth who cared about her

- Red Chestnut to help her to regain emotional independence. Many elderly people, living on their own with an animal companion, invest so much emotional energy into them that they suffer enormous pain when the animal dies.

Mary's progress on the remedies:

Mary underwent a rapid improvement some days after commencing the remedies. Her nihilistic thoughts and sense of waiting for death gradually gave way to a sense of brightness and hope, with the feeling that there could be some promise of potential happiness in this life. She stopped dwelling so much on upsetting memories, no longer lost in that rose-tinted daydream of a distant reunion with her lost ones. Her appetite improved and she was much more able to live in, and appreciate, the present moment.

After a few weeks taking her remedies, Mary telephoned Kate to say she wanted to come and visit. Kate was delighted at this change in her mother. Then, as they spoke on the phone, she heard the sound of barking in the background. 'What's that I hear?' she asked. Her mother said: 'Bill Junior!' She had gone to a local dog pound and picked out a six-month-old mongrel who closely resembled Bill. This was the breakthrough development in the case, showing clearly how Mary had become able to integrate the memory of Bill in a positive, healthy manner and was now able to look forward to the future. Bill Junior symbolised her desire to keep on living and to make the most out of life.

The action of Bach flower remedies on grief

A frequently asked question is 'what's a good remedy for grief?' Let's examine this question, and what it means.

It should be understood that grief, as the outpouring of pent-up sadness, isn't only a natural process but also a very necessary one. Grief should not be suppressed, and to seek a remedy 'for' grief, that that will eradicate the symptoms of grief – just stamping them out so as not to have to face them – is wrong-minded. We shouldn't wish to 'blank out' the feelings we have for someone we have cared for. In one sense, the grief we feel is a way of paying tribute to the departed loved one, remembering how important their presence was to us. Through positive grieving we honour the legacy they have left us, the impression they have made on our own lives, and what we can learn from them.

Yet it does hurt, and we need to address the sense of devastation and pain. Bach remedies don't act as an emotional analgesic in the manner of a sedative drug; instead they are able to help with the process of expressing, integrating and then releasing pain. Once the pain is released, we can move on to enjoy the bittersweet memory of happy times gone by whilst also enjoying the present moment and looking ahead to the future. The remedies allow us to draw a balance between darkness and light: we mourn, but life goes on. A fine example of a healthy mourning process is the old tradition of the 'wake', especially as seen in Irish culture where the memory of the departed was toasted with much festivity and partying. This gives a good idea of how the different poles of sorrow and joy, light and darkness, can actually be healthily brought together in grief.

Releasing the pain in this way helps to prevent the first acute or 'inflammatory' stage of grief from dragging on too long, or from becoming deeply entrenched as a bleeding wound in the mind. People who have been so affected by the death of a pet or other loved one that they go on for months or even years unable to get over the sadness, need to work through the trapped pain that is torturing them, so they can put it behind them and move forward. Bach flower remedies are an important way to help this vital process.

Chapter Six

Practicalities of giving Bach Remedies to Dogs

Bach flower remedies are easy to give to animals – and of all the animals that people keep as pets or companions, dogs are probably the easiest to give remedies to. Whilst cats tend to be a wee bit more discriminating about what they're offered to eat, domestic dogs with their scavenger origins will happily gobble up anything that's offered them without asking any questions. Their lack of fussiness makes our job of giving them remedies that bit easier!

A word of caution

Before we go on, there's one very important rule to remember. In fact, the following is the one and only safety caution involved in Bach flower therapy for animals. As you will have seen, Bach remedies come in small bottles with glass pipettes from which the drops are dispensed. The first and most important rule of giving Bach flower remedies to dogs (and other animals) and in fact the only safety caution in flower remedy therapy, is:

> *Never give drops direct from the dropper*
> *into a dog's mouth.*

This is simply due to the fact that the dropper tube is made of thin glass and could cause serious harm if bitten off and swallowed. Dogs can move very fast, and may snap at the dropper if they think it's something to eat. The authors have never, in many years' experience, heard of a case of a dog or any other animal being harmed in this way, but it's nonetheless very important to follow this safety rule.

Methods of administering Bach remedies to dogs

Bach remedies are usually (but not always) given by mouth. The easiest and most obvious way to do this is with a dog is by putting drops into a dog's food. How many drops should you give per day? Dr Bach described various methods of dosage, but the most normal dosage instructions with Bach remedies for people are to take about 4 drops, 4 times daily, either straight from the bottle or in a little water – so about 16 drops in all. The precise number of drops isn't vitally important, as long as the dosage is steady and consistent. As Dr Bach himself wrote:

> 'It does not matter about being exact, as none of these remedies could do the least harm, even if taken in large quantities, but as a little is enough, to make up a small amount saves waste.'
>
> (Collected Writings of Edward Bach)

Deciding how many drops to give a dog at a time depends on how often your dog eats. Many dogs, especially larger dogs, are given two meals a day, one in the morning and the other later in the day. In such a case, it's practical and effective to split the daily dose of 16 or so drops into two lots and give about 8 drops, twice daily with each meal. As with humans, there's no need to worry too much about dosage precision – the exact number of drops is less important than keeping up a good, steady and consistent dosage.

To give the drops this way, simply prepare the dog's dish with whatever food he eats – this should always be a good quality food that provides the dog with all the nourishment he needs – and then drop the drops on top of the food. They do not need to be absorbed.

Some dogs may be in the habit of rushing in to start eating before you've finished putting the drops on the food. This should be avoided, not simply because it's bad manners for the dog to act this way, but also because of the potential risk of the glass dropper being bitten before you get a chance to withdraw it. Make the dog wait for his food by training him to stand back until you release him with a command such as 'OK'. If your dog training skills aren't up to scratch, you could prepare the food on a kitchen worktop out of the dog's reach before placing the dish with added remedies on the floor for him.

If your dog only eats one meal a day, as is often the way with smaller breeds, you might wish to give half the daily drops with that meal and then give the rest in some other way. Drops can also be added to other types of food, other than the dog's regular meals. Many types of biscuit made for dogs are absorbent enough for you to be able to add a few drops of a flower remedy to them.

Using training snacks

Pieces of biscuit or dried food make good snacks to give to a dog as a reward in training: every time the dog does what you want him to do, he can have a reward. When he doesn't do what you want, he gets no reward. This way, you can make the dog work for his rewards, learn his lessons, and at the same time add drops to some of the snacks as a practical way of giving the dog Bach remedies. Small pieces of bread are also very absorbent and a good way to feed a few drops of remedy. Most dogs will eat them down without hesitation. Don't feed too much processed white bread to dogs, and only give them little bits to avoid choking them. Remember, it's very unhealthy for a dog to be even slightly overweight. If you're feeding a dog a number of treats, snacks and rewards during the day, cut down the size of his meals accordingly to make sure he isn't getting too much food.

Giving Bach remedies in drinking water

Dogs should always have a supply of fresh water available, and adding drops of remedies to drinking water is another way to give Bach remedies to dogs. It doesn't matter that the drops become more dilute by adding them to a bowl or dish of water. If Bach remedies were a traditional herbal remedy that works by the action of plant chemicals, diluting them this much would be a problem because it would weaken the concentration of chemicals and perhaps make them too weak to work. But due to the way Bach remedies work, dilution isn't a problem. If desired, you can add 8 drops twice daily, or 4 drops 4 times daily, to a dog's drinking water.

Too many dogs for one dish

The only practical problem with this approach is if you have more than one dog drinking out of the same water dish. Dogs are decidedly hierarchical creatures, and a higher-ranking dog may sometimes delight in monopolising the water dish to make a statement. (The authors' Rottweiler vainly tries to assert his leadership over our Pekingese this way, for instance – of course he's fooling nobody!) If this happens, the wrong dog might get the remedies and the dog you want to give them to might get too little or none!

But if you discover that Rover has lapped up all the water containing the remedies intended for Fido, don't panic. One of the greatest virtues of the Bach remedies, that really sets them apart from virtually all other plant-based natural therapies, is that they will only have an effect if they're needed. Giving the wrong remedies, or the right ones to the wrong dog, will simply have no effect at all. However, that's going to be of little consolation to the dog deprived of his remedies. You will have to find a solution to the problem. Giving the dogs separate water dishes, one with remedies and the other without, and hoping that they will drink out of the right ones, is probably expecting too much! You may find it's simply easier to give the drops in food instead. Another simple way to give Bach remedies orally to dogs is to simply place a few drops in your hand and let the dog lick them off.

Making a treatment bottle

Treatment bottles are a simple and practical way to:

1. Give several remedies at a time from the same bottle

2. Save on remedies… and on money!

3. Reduce alcohol content if desired

To make a treatment bottle, take an empty and clean dropper bottle (30ml is an ideal size, although 10ml will also do fine). Fill this bottle with fresh, clean water, preferably bottled mineral water (still, not sparkling). Add 2 or 3 drops of each remedy you want to use to the bottle, creating a tailor-made combination to suit the dog's requirements. Give it a little shake to mix up the contents and it's ready to use. Some people believe you should shake the bottle vigorously before each time you use it. Theoretically, this increases the 'potency' of the remedy very slightly, energising it by electrical friction; however it's not necessary to do this.

If you choose to add about 25% brandy or similar alcohol to preserve the water in the treatment bottle, at the normal dosage (of about 16 drops a day) a 30ml treatment bottle will last approximately 28 days. Alternatively, if you prefer to keep it alcohol-free, just keep the bottle stored in the fridge when not in use. The unpreserved water should last about 5 days, after which you can throw away any that's left over, and make another treatment bottle. Dosage from this treatment bottle is exactly as though you were using a 'normal' Bach remedy, about 4 drops 4 times or 8 drops twice daily. Again, don't worry about the extra stage of dilution, even when this diluted mixture is further diluted in water dishes. We are working with subtle energy here, not crude chemicals.

The wrong bottle!

A word of advice: don't forget to label treatment bottles, either with the name of the dog or with the names of the remedies! If you're giving Bach remedies to more than one dog in the household and you forget which treatment bottle is which, it'll be impossible to tell them apart. Alternatively, you could use bottles of different colour, e.g. a green one for Fido and an amber one for Rover... but it's probably easier just to obtain some of those cheap sticky office labels from your local stationer and scribble the dogs' names on them. Do remember, though, that if you should give the wrong remedy to the wrong dog by mistake, no harm can possibly occur.

Sprays

Extending the idea of the treatment bottle, you can use the same trick to make a spray bottle. Bach spray bottles are a very handy alternative to giving remedies by mouth. These are useful when:

1. Dogs are ill or unconscious and you're waiting for veterinary attention

2. Dogs are acting aggressively due to fear and can't be approached, e.g. rescue dogs in kennels

3. Dogs are nervous in the car and it's not feasible to stop and give them drops in food or water

4. Everyone in the household is a little stressed and needs some help

The mixture from a spray bottle will have exactly the same effect as usual. You simply pump a few puffs into the air around the dog. Tiny molecules of water containing the signature of the remedy will drift down; some land on the skin and are picked up by subtle electrical sensors, and others are inhaled into the system. When spraying, do not spray in the dog's eyes, nose or other sensitive areas. Spray over the dog's head and around his body, at least a foot away.

Empty spray bottles can be obtained cheaply. To make one up, simply fill with still mineral water and add 4-5 drops of whatever remedy or remedies you wish to use. If the spray is to be kept for a while and used regularly, either keep it in the fridge or add 15-20% brandy to it to preserve the water. Some people like to add 1 or 2 drops of an essential (aromatherapy) oil such as Lavender. This gives the spray a pleasant smell and some oils also have a relaxing effect (a chemical effect unlike the effect of the Bach remedies). Note: do not put too many drops of essential oil in, as an excessive amount of some oils can cause headaches and other problems. *Note: Adding essential oils also makes the spray mixture unsafe to use orally, as most essential oils are not suitable for internal use.*

Creams and lotions

The Bach mixture most often used on the skin in cream form is the classic combination of Impatiens, Cherry Plum, Star of Bethlehem, Clematis and Rock Rose, with the addition of Crab Apple. This enhanced 'rescue remedy' formula is available as Five-Flower Cream from Healing Herbs. It has many potential uses, including helping to heal burns and minor injuries, rashes and irritations, insect bites and inflammation. It has also been used to help dogs with flea-bite dermatitis, an allergic reaction that many dogs suffer from when they have been bitten by parasites. 5-Flower cream also contains almond oil and borax, which are known for their ability to help with skin problems.

You can also make a cream out of any combination of remedies you choose for any individual dog or particular problem. A few drops of one or more remedies can be mixed into jars of creams or lotions for rubbing onto the skin. A bland, neutral pH cream is needed for use on a dog's skin. Your home-made cream can then be used topically in just the same way.

Baths

Many owners – especially of smaller dogs which are more manageable – like to give their pets the occasional shampoo in the kitchen or utility room sink, or in the bath or shower if they prefer! A few drops of one or more remedies can be added to bath water to help relax dogs if they are a little stressed and anxious while being bathed. Note: dogs should not be bathed too often as this can strip away the natural skin and coat oils. Once every couple of months is enough. Only special dog shampoo products should be used. Vets generally recommend that young puppies should not be bathed at all.

The amazing acu-points

A surprisingly effective method of giving the remedies was first pioneered in Australia (by the Australasian Flower Essence Academy) and further developed for animal use by the Society for Animal Flower Essence Research. This fascinating method involves the use of a major cranial acu-point. This is an energy centre at the very top of the head, lying halfway between the ears of a dog (or cat, or horse). Energy centres around the body are the basis of therapies such as acupuncture, which are now scientifically tested and fast becoming part of mainstream medicine across the world. They are points where it seems we can connect with, or tap into, the many flows of subtle electrical bio-energy around the body.

Research has shown that topical application of flower remedy drops on this energy point on the head gives very effective results. Simply drop two or three drops of a remedy, or from a remedy combination in a treatment bottle, into the palm of your hand.

Gently smooth the liquid into the fur on the top of the dog's head, taking care not to let any of it run into the eyes. There's no need to rub the remedies into the skin, or for them to be absorbed. Ultra-sensitive receptor cells at the acu-point can detect the minute electrical signals from the remedy and 'read' the information. This method can be used several times each day just as one would do with oral doses.

The acu-point system has sometimes been known to be more effective than the more usual oral method of taking remedies. It also offers a brilliant advantage, in that it's perfect for giving drops to a dog that is sick, unconscious, or distressed. It avoids having to give the dog anything to eat or drink, which can be forbidden if the dog is due to have an operation in the next few hours. It's very simple and quick to wet your hand with a few drops and gently pat the dog's head. This can be done any time, for instance during training.

Whichever method you use, keep giving doses of the remedies regularly each day. Consistency is the most important thing. Because the remedies are subtle by nature, they need to be given a chance to work. In most normal situations, it will take more than a day or two to see results and just giving a few drops one day and then nothing for two days will tend to produce poor results.

Giving remedies in an emergency situation

When giving remedies to a dog for acute shock, trauma, terror, or at a time of emergency, flower remedies can be given more frequently than the normal dosage. Drops may be given as necessary, perhaps every few minutes until the animal starts to calm down. Many people will use 5-Flower Formula as a general 'emergency remedy' in such situations. This is often very fast-acting and, by keeping up a steady dosage of a few drops every few minutes, it's often possible to calm a distressed animal.

If in doubt, or if you think the dog is injured or in pain, call the vet immediately. Dogs that have become suddenly uncontrollable or aggressive for no apparent reason may have something wrong with them that requires urgent veterinary attention, and in these cases do not try to use flower remedies as a replacement for medical care.

If the dog is very frightened or in distress he may well not be interested in food or water at this moment. DO NOT try to put the drops straight into his mouth with the glass dropper, as this is inviting disaster. You could use a soft plastic syringe to get the drops in, or else simply rub some of the remedy by hand into the dog's gums and tongue, taking care not to get bitten if the dog is in distress. Alternatively use the acu-point method as described above, simply wetting the top of the dog's head with liberal quantities of the remedies until you can hand him over to the vet. Don't forget to keep taking drops yourself – if you can spare them – in order to keep a clear head during an emergency situation.

Chapter Seven

Frequently-asked Questions

In this chapter we'll recap on some of the points made in the book by setting out some of the most frequently-asked questions about Bach flower remedies and dogs.

Question 1: How safe are Bach remedies to give to my dog?

If you've read the book, you already know the answer. However, let's remind ourselves again as it's such an important point: Bach remedies are very, very safe. They can be given to all dogs, from the very young to the very elderly. They are safe to give to pregnant females or sick animals undergoing veterinary treatment. Not a single adverse reaction has ever been recorded with this type of remedy in over 70 years. They are hypoallergenic, drug and chemical free. It's theoretically impossible to cause any problems by 'overdosing' as the remedies are so safe and gentle in their action. If you give a remedy that isn't needed by the dog, the active constituents will simply fail to act. As Dr Bach himself said:

> 'As all the remedies are pure and harmless, there is no fear of giving too much or too often, though only the smallest quantities are necessary to act as a dose. Nor can any remedy do harm should it prove not to be the one actually needed for the case.'
>
> (Collected writings of Edward Bach)

Question 2: I want to give my dog Bach remedies, but he's on conventional medication. Is that OK?

This is an important question, as so many dogs (like people) are receiving medication for one problem or another. Some herbal remedies can cause problems if given to a dog that is on medical drugs. These problems are called drug interactions, caused by the reaction of chemicals together. Such drug interactions can also be problem when one medical drug reacts with another, and with certain types of food. Doctors and vets (in theory, at least) are careful not to allow patients to suffer the negative effects of drug interactions.

But because the Bach flower remedies don't contain chemicals or rely on chemicals for their therapeutic action, these drug interactions can't happen. This means that the remedies can't interfere with medical drugs. Bach flower remedies are also perfectly suited for use alongside other types of medicine, such as herbal or homeopathic medicine. Whatever you use or the vet prescribes for your dog, you can use the Bach remedies freely. This is a very important and valuable property of flower remedies, which isn't found in many other effective natural therapies.

In many cases, using flower remedies alongside conventional medicine has not only proven to be safe, but has also helped the animal to need less of the conventional medicine by gently promoting a happier, healthier animal. This is especially true if dogs and other animals have been suffering from physical problems as a result of stress: for instance skin problems that have come on due to emotional tension and are not too deeply established as chronic diseases in their own right. As long as the disease has not gained too strong a grip, and if the dog's immune system is reasonably healthy, helping to make the dog more relaxed mentally can gradually help the disease to be eliminated. This is such an important step for an unfortunate dog that is already suffering stress but is also afflicted by the toxic damage of long-term medication with drugs such as steroids, which vets often give out much too easily with little knowledge of potential side effects.

Question 3: Why do the Bach remedies contain so much alcohol? Is that what makes them work, and is it toxic in any way?

The medium that carries the healing qualities of the Bach remedies is ordinary H2O, plain water. Unfortunately, water doesn't remain fresh on its own, and unless preserved somehow it becomes a breeding ground for bacteria. Commercial Bach flower producers have mainly used alcohol – either grape alcohol or brandy, sometimes vodka – to preserve the water.

The alcohol content of the remedies in no way contributes to their effect. This can be demonstrated in different ways: firstly, the remedies still work when greatly diluted; secondly, they still work when given topically as opposed to orally; they work in sprays when they don't come into contact with the dog at all. Moreover, if the alcohol were having the effect, there would be nothing to differentiate one remedy from the other, and they would all work the same! The fact that giving the 'wrong' remedy will fail to have an effect tends to contradict this idea.

Are there any health risks giving animals remedies containing alcohol? If we were giving dogs any significant quantity of the remedies, the answer to this would probably be yes. However, due to the very tiny amounts involved if you adhere to the proper dosage routine, it's extremely unlikely that even over a period of years the alcohol content of the drops could have any significant toxic effect. There has never been any known case of this happening. If, however, you are concerned about the alcohol content of the remedies as they come straight from the bottle you purchase from your supplier, you can reduce the quantity of alcohol very significantly by making a treatment bottle as described in the previous chapter.

Question 4: How long do the remedies take to work?

In most cases of Bach flower therapy, assuming that the problem is a case for Bach remedies in the first place, and that the right remedies have been selected and properly administered, results are usually seen within two to three weeks, and sometimes much sooner than that. Naturally, results depend on the individual dog and the nature and severity of the problem for which he's being treated.

Interestingly, practice has shown that milder types of problems, such as everyday fears and anxiety, can take a little longer, perhaps two weeks or so, to be helped. Meanwhile, more severe and acute problems such as shock, strong fears and the severe anxiety of rescue dogs with a history of being beaten and maltreated, can often take much less time to react to the Bach remedies. Therapists and owners have often seen very frightened, nervous or fearfully aggressive dogs become calmer within just a few minutes, as few as 4 or 5 minutes. Remedies such as Star of Bethlehem and Rock Rose seem to be very important for gaining these fast and spectacular results. Remedies like Mimulus, which are for milder types of fear, generally do not work as fast. So, strangely enough, we can often predict that the highly traumatised, battered and abused rescue dog will show positive responses to the remedies sooner and more obviously than the relatively less stressed family pet. The same curious effect seems to apply to human Bach flower therapy: often, the worse the problem, the faster and better the effect of the remedies. A person suffering from terrible grief or despair can often respond sooner than a person with mild anxiety.

Question 5: How many remedies can I combine together at a time?

It's only very occasionally that you will only need to use just one Bach remedy on its own. In most situations, you will need to use two or more, and sometimes quite a few together. In fact, it's perfectly all right to use up to 6 or 8 remedies at a time.

As for what would be the *maximum* effective number of remedies to combine together, in truth nobody has ever really been able to establish this. One reason is that it wouldn't be ethical to deliberately give 20 remedies together to a traumatised dog to see whether they would still work. In such situations, you just get on with the business of helping the animal and leave scientific curiosity aside! In any case, it's not really important to establish a maximum number, whether it be 12, 15, 25 or 30 remedies, as it's normally (always, in our experience) possible to whittle the choice of remedies down to around 6 or 7.

Question 6: How long can I go on using the remedies? Are they OK for long-term use?

Because they're so safe, the Bach remedies are perfectly viable for long-term use if necessary. You can go on using Bach flower remedies for as long as required, and until you see their benefits firmly established and the problem as much helped as it can be. Because the remedies can't cause toxicity, it's impossible to overdose. Nor will pets become 'used' to their effect and require increasing doses to get the benefit, as can happen with drug-based treatments.

When people see their dogs and other animals responding well to Bach remedies, their next question is often 'will I have to keep my dog on these remedies forever?' The answer is that, even if this should be necessary, it can't do any harm. In practice, however, it's usually not necessary to give the remedies for extended periods as they can have a very deep-acting curative effect.

For deeper problems, especially where the emotional problem is mixed up with a lot of learned behaviours (for instance in attention-seeking problems in dogs), it may be wise to keep up the dosage of the remedies for a good period of time, perhaps several months. Even when you see the problem helped, keep the remedies going for a while to make sure that the effect is well established.

Any necessary changes to the remedy formula/combination can be made at any time, allowing you to conduct an intelligent, well-structured and effective course of therapy.

Question 7: Can Bach flower remedies help with physical problems?

Yes and no. In his writings Dr Bach made the rather bold claim that all disease was caused by negative emotions, and that once these problems were helped, all disease would just vanish. It would be wonderful if it were true; however, Dr Bach's idea should be taken with a large pinch of salt, as it isn't really borne out in practice.

So how far can Bach remedies help with physical illness? In lighter cases, when stress is causing minor physical problems that appeared relatively recently and haven't become chronic, there's no doubt that Bach remedies can have a very good indirect effect on the physical level. For instance, many owners report that acute anxiety-related problems like colitis can be helped by using flower remedies. Research has shown that in many cases helping an animal on an emotional/psychological level to feel happier and less stressed can also have an indirect effect on physical health. We also know that Bach remedies have sometimes been reported to have a marked effect on certain physical problems, such as

Scleranthus in helping with hormonal swings in bitches, when given for associated emotional problems.

However, in more serious cases of disease and in cases where the physical problem isn't stress-related, Bach flower remedies are really out of their jurisdiction and should not be considered the appropriate approach. Certain remedies like Gorse, Mustard, Olive or Wild Rose can be of complementary use in helping to boost an animal's vitality when ill. Animals that are very fearful due to their problem may also be helped. But the flower remedies will not provide the complete solution, by any means.

Even problems that were originally stress-related but have gone on to become very chronic might not respond well to Bach remedies. For instance, ex-rescue dogs that have suffered immune system weakness and chronic disease as a result of severe, prolonged stress in the past can benefit from Bach flower therapy for emotional and behavioural problems, but the remedies should not be relied on to treat their physical illnesses. We all want to use natural remedies as much as is practical with our animals, and wish to avoid the use of conventional medicines for them, if possible. However, if a pet is ill, home use of natural remedies should not be considered as an alternative to seeking veterinary help.

Question 8: I'm interested in using Bach remedies for my dog but I need to know that I can trust them. Do healthcare professionals such as vets and doctors recommend or use these remedies?

Yes, in many countries such professionals are using these types of remedies increasingly often, drawn to them for their simplicity of use, absolute safety record and high success rate. In Britain and the USA there are many veterinarians who favour Bach remedies as well as related therapies such as homeopathy. Associations such as the British Association of Homeopathic Veterinary Surgeons are growing all the time and promoting the use of these safe and effective approaches.

The Growth of Flower Remedy and other Complementary Therapy in the Mainstream – some facts:

- 30% of doctors in Denmark and Germany use flower remedies and other complementary therapies.

- As part of the growth of natural therapies in the mainstream, 20% of veterinary surgeries in the UK use herbal remedies

- The Cuban Ministry of Public Health invited two Professors from Argentina to teach the first official course in flower remedy therapy to doctors and other medical professionals in 1997. By October 1998 there were 104 graduates, with 25 research studies showing notable results in treating various physical and psychological pathologies such as migraines, depression, skin conditions, menopausal symptoms, stress and asthma. Due to these encouraging results, the authorities at the Ministry of Public Health officially recognised flower remedies in January 1999 as a valid medical modality to be integrated into the National Health System.

- Several scientific trials conducted by doctors in the USA and Central America have demonstrated significant reductions in depression on both the Beck and Hamilton Depression Inventories after flower remedy therapy.

- In Australia, flower remedy therapy is now being used in many major hospitals. One of its uses has been in special pain management units, helping with mental tension and resulting muscular tension and pain in patients recovering from major surgery who could not obtain full relief from opiate drugs.

- In Australia it is now also possible to take a University degree in flower remedy studies, and thanks to the pioneering work of the Australasian Flower Essence Academy (later renamed the LiFE Academy) flower remedies were successfully introduced into many Australian hospitals for use in special pain management centres.

- Adverse effects from the use of flower remedy therapy are unknown and have never emerged either in anecdotal reports or in scientific studies.

Chapter Eight

Bach Flower Remedy Combinations

The following are some suggested ideas for ready-made combinations, geared to suit specific situations and purposes. Following the instructions on how to make a treatment bottle, it's simple and straightforward to make your own combinations, or 'combos', up at home. By adding about 25% brandy or similar alcohol, it's then possible to keep the combos stored, ready for immediate use, for months. You can also add a new remedy to a combo at any time, allowing you to experiment to find the best recipe to suit an individual dog. As your expertise grows, you can very easily add to the list below, creating effective combinations of your own for any number of situations.

Post-Operation Combo

To help a dog to recuperate psychologically from an operation:

Clematis / Gentian / Impatiens / Oak / Olive / Rock Rose / Star of Bethlehem / Wild Rose

Show Combo

To help a dog that is stressed, nervous or confused at a show, and who becomes exhausted or overwhelmed by excitement:

Cherry Plum / Clematis / Elm / Impatiens / Larch / Mimulus / Olive / Rock Rose / Star of Bethlehem / Walnut

Vitality Combo

A general aid to boosting energy and vitality:

Elm / Hornbeam / Mustard / Oak / Olive / Wild Rose

Rescue Dog

To help with a range of problems associated with past trauma or any negative experiences a dog may have suffered that are causing emotional problems in the present:

Beech / Mimulus / Mustard / Rock Rose / Star of Bethlehem / Wild Rose

Bereavement Combo

To help dogs that are suffering from the loss of a companion or friend, human or animal:

Gentian / Gorse / Honeysuckle / Mustard / Star of Bethlehem / Walnut / Wild Rose

Training Combo

To help sharpen cognitive skills, learning ability and concentration:

Chestnut Bud / Clematis / Impatiens / Larch / Rock Water / Vervain

Travel Combo

For stress problems associated with car travel:

Cherry Plum / Elm / Impatiens / Rock Rose / Scleranthus / Star of Bethlehem / Walnut

New Pup Combo (for the pup)

To help a puppy settle into his new home and adapt to the unfamiliar environment as well as to aid socialisation:

Elm / Honeysuckle / Larch / Mimulus / Star of Bethlehem / Walnut / Water Violet

New Pup Combo (for the older dog)

To help other dogs in the household adapt more easily to any social upheaval caused by the arrival of the new pack member:

Beech / Holly / Larch / Vine / Walnut / Water Violet / Willow

Pack Harmony Combo

A general aid to creating a harmonious social environment for all the dogs in the household. This could be given separately to each dog or used in a spray:

Beech / Cherry Plum / Holly / Water Violet / Willow

Veteran Combo

To help older dogs with some of the common emotional problems they may suffer, such as loss of confidence:

Aspen / Gorse / Larch / Mimulus / Olive / Star of Bethlehem / Walnut / Wild Rose

Chapter Nine

Case Histories
from the S.A.F.E.R. Archives

Buttons

Mrs Williams of Cardiff, UK, had a problem with her dog, an elderly Yorkshire terrier named Buttons. Buttons had undergone an operation and was suffering from what is often called the 'never been well since' syndrome. He started becoming very anxious and fearful at night, and was disrupting Mrs Williams' sleep. The dog was also becoming increasingly afraid of thunder, going into severe states of terror at the slightest storm. Unfortunately, it was a stormy time of year and he was being very badly affected. A friend told Mrs Williams about the Society for Animal Flower Essence Research, S.A.F.E.R for short, and she called for some advice. With guidance she was able to choose some remedies to suit Buttons' problem.

The remedies chosen were the Bach flower remedies Larch (to help promote the dog's confidence), Mimulus (to help dispel fear and anxiety), Rock Rose (to address more acute and pressing states of severe fear), and Star of Bethlehem (to address the trauma of the operation, which had apparently been the trigger for his emotional decline).

The drops were fed to Buttons in his food, eight drops twice daily. Results were seen very rapidly. The remedies were obtained on a Friday and Mrs Williams called the following Monday to report positive changes. On the Friday night, Buttons had slept much better than usual, only wakening her up once at around 6am. The following night he slept soundly without any disturbance at all. On the Sunday afternoon, the third day on the drops, there was a huge thunderstorm. Instead of displaying his usual terror, Buttons slept through the storm very contentedly. He never looked back, and even though Mrs Williams only gave him the remedies for a month or so, the effect has been lasting: in over eighteen months the fear has not returned.

The case of the sad little stray

S.A.F.E.R dog behaviour expert Sandra Morris was contacted by a lady who had recently found a small, emaciated and trembling dog on her doorstep. The dog had evidently been abandoned, and prior to that, badly abused and tortured: it bore the marks of cigarette burns and other cruel wounds. A vet had dealt with the physical problems but the dog's worst problems were emotional, after such an unimaginable ordeal. The lady wanted to see Sandra immediately, to gain her expert advice on how to get the dog to trust again and bond with her. The dog was so terrified of humans that it was spending most of its time cringing behind furniture.

Sandra, unfortunately, had a full schedule that meant she couldn't see the dog immediately. She explained this to the desperate owner but suggested that in the meantime she could try giving the dog some Star of Bethlehem. The lady was willing to try anything safe to help the dog, and she purchased some immediately. When Sandra arrived for the consultation a week or so later, the lady opened the door and to Sandra's surprise, a happy little dog with a wagging tail jumped up to greet her. The owner was crying, not with sadness but with joy. This was the same dog that only a few days before had been so frightened that it would approach nobody. Sandra's expertise was needed to take the dog further and teach it some lead work; however, she told us that without the help of the flower remedies she believed that this dog could never have come so far.

Jacques

This is the case of a Retriever named Jacques who lives in France. His owner, Marie, sensed something was wrong when Jacques suddenly developed a strong fear of travelling in the car. He would no longer even approach the car voluntarily and was very unwilling to get inside. He could be lured in with titbits, but this did not always work and it took a long time. Once the engine was started and the car began to move, he would 'freak out' completely. Prior to this he had always been a good traveller.

Jacques was checked by his vet and given the all-clear. The vet couldn't explain the new behaviour.

Marie knew about the Bach Flower Remedies and tried giving the dog Mimulus (for fears and anxieties) and Rock Rose (for acute terror), four drops four times daily on pieces of dried bread or biscuit. This produced a slight result after two weeks, but Jacques' fear would still return as soon as the car engine was started. Marie would have to stop the car and console him. At this point she contacted S.A.F.E.R for help.

The first thing that the therapists advised was that Marie should stop petting Jacques when he showed fear. This was an understandable reaction from a loving and concerned owner, but was tending to reinforce his fear by rewarding him at the moment of the frightening stimulus. A classic behavioural mistake that many owners make! The second point was to ask Marie whether anything had sparked this condition – had anything happened in the car, such as a minor accident or other frightening incident? Marie couldn't think of any, and for the moment the cause of Jacques' problem remained a mystery.

Mimulus and Rock Rose, having been mildly effective with him, were continued, and a new remedy added to the mix: Star of Bethlehem, the remedy that addresses all manner of past traumatic incidents and their imprint on the mind. We felt that some kind of traumatic, frightening experience must be the unseen cause of the problem. These three remedies were administered to the dog as before, with the strict understanding that any displays of fear from Jacques were to be ignored and not rewarded. After one week, the dog was happy to sit in the car for short trips. After ten days, he was fine on a longer trip. Since that time (the case was taken in early 2001) there has been no repetition of the problem.

It later transpired that just before Jacques' problem started, Marie's 19-year-old son, whilst home on vacation from college, had taken him out in the car, driving without his mother's permission. He had been speeding, and narrowly avoided a serious accident. The experience had left him very shaken, but he had not told his mother about it. Here was the missing piece of the puzzle! This was the 'unseen' trauma that had triggered the dog's fearful behaviour, explaining why the first two remedies given had not completely eased his stress. It was necessary to heal the frightening memory of the near-accident, the panic and fright of his human companion.

This case showed that, as long as one is able to make educated guesses, flower remedy therapy allows us to treat problems without even having to know the details. This is another tribute to the amazing flexibility of the remedies.

Appendix – Resources

Bach flower remedy suppliers:

Healing Herbs Ltd
P.O Box 65, Hereford, HR2 0UW, UK
Tel: 01873 890218
www.healing-herbs.co.uk
Healing Herbs Ltd produce the full range of Bach remedies as well as Five-Flower Cream. These remedies are made in strict accordance with the original method used by Dr Bach and are unsurpassed for their quality and the attention to detail that goes into their preparation.

Ainsworths Homeopathic Pharmacy
36 New Cavendish Street, London W1M 7LH
Tel: +44 (0)207 935 5330
www.ainsworths.com
Ainsworths supply the full range of Bach remedies as well as a wide variety of homeopathic remedies.

Tortue Rouge Ltd
Tortue Rouge produce a range of specially-designed combinations of Bach flower remedies for animals, helping with problems including separation anxiety, show nerves, past abuse, general fears and anxiety, and bereavement. The remedies, called Dr Petals' Elixirs, are 100% organic and have been found very effective in many cases.
Tel: 0871 9008544
www.tortuerouge.co.uk

Readers in the USA can obtain the 38 Bach remedies from:

The Flower Essence Society (FES)
P.O Box 459, Nevada City, CA 95959
Tel: 800-736-9222
www.flowersociety.org

Neals Yard Remedies
Neals Yard is based in the UK and distributes Bach flower remedies to many countries of the world.
Tel/Fax: +44 (0) 161 8317875
www.nealsyardremedies.com

Canine diets

As mentioned in the book, diet is an important factor in a dog's behaviour and general state of health and happiness. Some cases of 'hyperactivity' in dogs are in fact due to dietary causes, and some veterinary experts have linked uncontrollable behaviour, even aggression, to certain inappropriate diets. It's important to realise that while one dog might thrive on a certain diet, another may not. Some dog breeds have quite specific requirements, and individual dogs of the same breed may not always do well on the same food. There is probably no one food that is perfect for all, and so a certain amount of experimentation is usually needed to find what suits your own dog or dogs. It's important to avoid cheap and low-quality diets, as many of these will simply not provide adequate nutrition and this is bound to affect health. Below are three recommended UK brands that, although commercial, are of good quality.

- **NatureDiet** – soft cooked meat, comes in a range of varieties packed in 390g tubs. Contact: 08700 132960 / www.naturediet.co.uk

- **Burns** – dried kibble-type food of high quality, developed by a vet with a lifelong interest in holistic health; there is also an organic variety. Contact: +44 (0)1554 890482 / www.burns-pet-nutrition.co.uk

- **James Wellbeloved** – also a dried kibble-type, of a similar standard of quality as Burns. Available from most good pet supplies stores.

Books

Below are some recommended books for those wishing to learn more about dog behaviour problems, their causes and cures.

Think Dog

John Fisher, Blandford Books

Probably the first mainstream canine behaviour book ever to mention the Bach remedies. The late John Fisher was a truly pioneering dog behaviour expert who recognised that the real solution to most problems lay beyond the realm of traditional dog training methods.

Don't Dope the Dog

Martin J. Scott and Gael Mariani, S.A.F.E.R Publications

Tel: +44 (0)1267 281761

Email: dontdopethedog@uku.co.uk

This little book examines the scandal surrounding the use of psychotropic drugs such as Prozac and Valium in canine behaviour therapy and explores some safer, more effective alternatives including the Bach flower remedies, other flower remedies and homeopathy. Also available from Sheila Harper Canine Education: contact Erica Bennett on +44 (0) 1543 270026 / info@quanuk.com.

The Practical Dog Listener

Jan Fennell, HarperCollins

This sequel to the best-selling book The Dog Listener *is a practical handbook showing the application of Jan Fennell's simple and effective methods, expertly designed to reduce stress levels in dogs and help to eradicate unwanted behaviour.*

Canine behaviour organisations

The UK Canine and Feline Behaviour Association (CFBA) is one of the leading canine behaviour practices and teaching centres in the world and is highly recommended to readers wishing to consult a pet behaviourist for any type of problem. CFBA advocate only the most effective and gentle methods and are vociferously opposed to the growing tendency for vets and certain canine behaviourists to recommend the use of powerful mind-altering drugs for animal behaviour problems.

CFBA also co-produce a range of excellent self-help videos, designed to empower dog owners to tackle many common behaviour problems in their dogs, including separation anxiety, attention-seeking and aggression. The films are written and presented by CFBA Chairman Colin Tennant, one of the world's top canine behaviour experts, and are available on VHS or DVD.

The Canine and Feline Behaviour Association
Tel: +44 (0)1442 842374
www.cfba.co.uk

Jan Fennell
Jan Fennell is one of the world's foremost dog behaviour experts and the author of several best-selling books including The Dog Listener. *Jan Fennell gives consultations in the UK and runs training courses in Amichien Bonding, her own special and effective range of techniques for creating healthy relationships between people and their dogs. The Amichien method can be a very helpful adjunct to Bach flower therapy for dogs.*
Tel: +44 (0) 1724 761764
www.janfennellthedoglistener.com

Mary Lynne Doleys Amichien Bonding
Mary Lynne Doleys is a graduate of Jan Fennell's methods operating in the USA.
Skokie, IL USA
Tel: 1-224-210-0201
www.peacefulpaws.us
Email: info@peacefulpaws.us

Veterinary Associations

British Association of Homeopathic Veterinary Surgeons
Chinham House, Stanford-in-the-Vale, Nr. Faringdon
Oxfordshire, UK SN7 8NQ
Tel: 01367 710324
www.bahvs.com

American Holistic Veterinary Medical Association
2218 Old Emmorton Road
Bel Air, MD 21025
Tel: 1-410-569-0795
www.altvetmed.com

Education

The Animal Care College
Tel: +44 (0)1344 628269
www.animalcarecollege.co.uk
*Established for over 20 years, this specialist academy offers a wide variety of certificated and Open College Network-accredited home study courses in various aspects of animal care, including **Complementary Therapies for Pets** and **Bach Flower Remedies in Canine Care**.*

The Society for Animal Flower Essence Research (S.A.F.E.R)
Tel: +44 (0)1267 281761
Email: accnews@uku.co.uk
*S.A.F.E.R works in conjunction with its sister organisation The Natural Petcare Academy to provide a range of quality distance-learning courses in natural animal healthcare. S.A.F.E.R's flagship course is the highly-regarded **Diploma in Flower Essences for Animals** (Dip.FEA), offering practitioner-level training by distance in Bach flower remedies and other flower (and gem) essences for animals. The Dip.FEA course is available to students all around the world and is still, to our knowledge, the only authoritative course in existence offering this kind of training, at a competitive price.*